BLEEDER

BLEEDER

A Memoir

Shelby Smoak

Michigan State University Press
East Lansing

⊚The paper used in this publication meets the minimum requirements of ANSI/NISO Z39.48-1992 (R 1997) (Permanence of Paper).

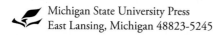 Michigan State University Press
East Lansing, Michigan 48823-5245

Printed and bound in the United States of America.

19 18 17 16 15 14 13   1 2 3 4 5 6 7 8 9 10

LIBRARY OF CONGRESS CATALOGING-IN-PUBLICATION DATA

Smoak, Shelby.
    Bleeder : a memoir / Shelby Smoak.
      p. cm.
    ISBN 978-1-60917-355-5 (ebook)—ISBN 978-1-61186-069-6 (pbk. : alk. paper) 1.
    Smoak, Shelby. 2. Hemophiliacs—Virginia—Biography. I. Title.
    RC642.S66 2013
    616.1'5720092—dc23
    [B]2012029287

Book design by Scribe Inc. (www.scribenet.com)
Cover design by David Drummond, Salamander Design, www.salamanderhill.com

Michigan State University Press is a member of the Green Press Initiative and is committed to developing and encouraging ecologically responsible publishing practices. For more information about the Green Press Initiative and the use of recycled paper in book publishing, please visit www.greenpressinitiative.org.

Visit Michigan State University Press at www.msupress.org

To my fellow hemophiliacs and HIV sufferers

At the end of my suffering
there was a door.

—LOUISE GLÜCK

CONTENTS

BLEEDER

BLOOD

I AM CAUCASIAN, FIVE FOOT ELEVEN, HAVE SANDY BROWN HAIR, BLUE eyes, and am a tender slip of bone. And I am at the hospital.

I am here because I have hemophilia; because my blood fails to clot normally; because I was a boy who received a defective X chromosome from his mother. Of course, it is not her fault, for until I was born, she didn't know she carried the defect. In fact, I am the only proof of it.

In 1974 when I was two, an unusually large bruise developed across my back and refused to heal. My parents were confused. How can this be? This bruise isn't normal? What is wrong with our son? Necessarily, their concern carried them (and me) to the emergency room—a site that will become commonplace to me as I age. Three days later, a test returned positive for hemophilia and my problem was solved. I was treated with a plasma product; the bruise healed; but I went home a hemophiliac, a free-bleeder. And my life changed forever.

Today, I am here for my six-month check up. Dr. Trum flips through my chart and jots notations as I wait. He is middle-aged, smart, and understands hemophilia from a very technical and scientific point of view. His face is broad and long, his nose large and bulbous and reddened along the snout, and he wears Buddy Holly glasses with black, pointed rims. They are his most noticeable characteristic and front a pale face and its white hair while the eyes behind the thick glass crease at the corners and underneath and are, as I imagine it, a result of long hours of medical study and, more recently, the worry and concern HIV has brought him. He clutches his clipboard, rustles my papers, makes another mark before he addresses me.

"You're eighteen now." My birthday passed five days ago. Then, Mom baked the cake; Dad and my sisters—Louise and Anne—sang the song. "So, I have to tell you the results of your HIV test," the doctor says.

I understand that the hemophiliacs were drastically affected by the tainted blood supply in the 1980s, and I think I intuited then how it would one day involve me, but I wasn't ready then for this kind of confrontation. I was just a child really. I recall sitting with Mom and Dad after the dinner meal one evening. I was attending high school, was perhaps a freshman or sophomore, and I suppose, too, that Anne and Louise had eaten and left the table, for I don't remember them being a part of this discussion. Dad folded his napkin underneath his plate and looked to Mom, who began the question.

"Son," she said, "have you been reading the papers and magazines and following the news about this HIV and AIDS?"

I nodded that I had.

"Then you know that the hemophiliacs are one of the risk groups."

Again, I answered yes.

"Then I wonder if you want to know about yourself. You were tested last year and your father and I know those results."

"You're in high school now," Dad interrupted. "It might be time you knew."

"But he's still just a kid, Shelby," Mom retorted to Dad. I looked at them as they looked at each other. Mom blew her nose in her napkin, wiped her face. Dad reached out his hand to cover Mom's trembling one. And then I shut out my fear.

"I don't want to know," I asserted.

Now, childhood can no longer shelter me.

"If you have to tell me, then tell me. What choice have I?"

"In 1985," Dr. Trum says, placing a hesitant finger to his glasses, "your test came back positive."

I am numb. I do not move.

My stomach twists, tightens. My body churns, knots, convulses. And my poached heart weeps its funerary rhythm.

My parents have kept this from me as I'd requested. And I realize now how their already hard-worn hearts must have torn with sadness all these years as I grew up. They protected me by their silence, like Trappists, saying prayers but not speaking. But today it changes. My innocence is shed from me. I am an adult. I am educated to grief and pain and hurt and death.

My life leaks out of me. Dr. Trum's voice becomes like a muffled drum. It throbs in my ears, but is lost as the hollow echo of the vacuum into which I have slunk. The doctor lays me out. He rustles his icy stethoscope against my expiring breath, and he rummages his cold hands along my frail bones. He tests the flex of my knee, the turn of my ankles, the sound of my breath, the beat of my plundered heart.

"How long have I had this?"

"Well," he says, returning to his desk and needling my file of papers. "Most of the infections occurred prior to 1984 before blood screening began." It is now 1990, I think as Dr. Trum pauses, resumes. "We can't say for sure at this point, but it's likely you were infected in the early eighties," pauses again, "if not before." It is all matter-of-fact for him and I hate that about him. Hate him. Hate his hospital clinic.

When I can think of anything amid this horror, it is of my grandmother. She is all I know of death. When we visited, she would sneak me cups of sweet coffee, and we would sip our brew in her parlor as the sun stole darkness from the morning. We would both smile at something secret and special we shared. And when she died, that notion was replaced by something blank as I tried, at eleven, to understand what it meant to pass away.

"How long do I have?" I ask. Yet I don't want an answer. I don't want my life bridled by a number.

Dr. Trum rambles, recounts statistics, offers hope, but shies from my question. I am no longer here. I am in a castle, in my thoughts. When I was a child dealing with my hemophilia, I relied upon this fantasy world, and my castles protected me then; its sorcery was my salvation. It was easy to imagine other worlds with kings and queens who ruled happily, knights and paladins that jousted gold-hungry dragons, and powerful mages whose shriveled hands healed and destroyed with intangible thought. And I try to conjure the magic of that place. This, however, is harder to defeat with fantasy. HIV is not a battle wound Merlin would understand.

"We want to get you started on AZT," Dr. Trum says.

"You do?"

"Yes. AZT will help stop HIV's spread."

I am handed a slip of prescription paper and ushered back to the lobby where Mom waits for me. As I near, she closes her magazine and I can read her sad and knowing look.

"Did they tell you?" she asks, rising slowly. Her whisper-fine strands of brown hair curl gently at her shoulders while her deep blue eyes sparkle in the flat, muffled hospital light.

"Yes."

"Are you okay?"

"I don't know, but I have to go to the pharmacy."

"Yes. But are you okay?"

"I have to go to the pharmacy."

We walk quietly down the crowded corridor. White coats hasten by us, and wheelchairs slow our speed. I pass the prescription to the pharmacist. I wait.

I have been here so many times for so many different prescriptions: the factor to replace the blood-clotting agent I lack; needles, syringes, and alcohol swabs for infusion; Amacar to decrease my bleeding during dental procedures; Ace bandages for my elbows, knees, and ankles; and so on. But this time is different. It is true that without the blood product for my hemophilia, I would have probably perished some time ago, but when I came in the past for factor prescriptions, I did not feel as threatened then as I do now. I accepted hemophilia as treatable. But HIV cannot offer me this. HIV feels as all the weight there is in the world. And its publicity causes all to fear it, even me. It is the plague of the 1980s and 1990s. And now I've got it.

The pharmacist looks to me, spinning the white bottle in his palms. My heart beats unsteadily. My hands shake and sweat. My breath labors as if my chest is gripped in a vice.

"Take one pill twice a day," he advises. "Morning and evening, and with meals. Any questions?"

"No."

"Okay. *Next.*"

And he slips the AZT in the bag, as simple as that.

On the two-hour ride home from Chapel Hill, I watch the scenery blur by on Highway 64. It changes quickly from university hospitals and giant building complexes to farms, barns, and ranch-style homes. The few cows not resting under shade trees cool themselves in the warm water of shallow ponds, dotting the red ponds and the red earth we pass by while the extreme heat causes a vapor to rise along the straight stretches of road. Mom cools the car with the air conditioning, and its mechanical blow and the flap of the car tire on hot asphalt gives a steady sound to our troubled ride. There are no cities near me and my knowledge of HIV is married to the cities, to things far away. I can't understand HIV's coming to me, sneaking into my blood under the guise of help as it did. For this, there is no answer, and will never be.

My mother and I are silent. The road we are on leads to the home that will never feel the same and the town that can never be the town it was to me before. I already feel dead.

Mom wheels into our driveway and I notice that in our front yard, the cherry tree no longer boasts vibrant purple-pink flowers but is green and wilted from the heat, and the dogwoods that corner our lot have folded their resurrection palms, have given way to the sweltering heat. They wilt and slink their once-supple branches in a weak, weeping hang.

That night, I eat a solemn and quiet dinner with my family. Little is spoken about my doctor's visit, but its tragedy is understood, our understanding made manifest in our muteness. Later, I fill a glass in my bathroom faucet and prepare to take my first dose of AZT, the inconspicuous white and blue pill that rolls so naturally in my hand. It is like any of the other pills I've taken, but it's the hardest one to swallow; it is only a temporary healing potion.

I go to my room, flip on my stereo, and realize it's the first time I've been alone with my HIV, and I'm not sure what to do with all the quiet. Not comfortable in my bed, I move to a chair and pretend I'm reading a book;

on the floor I play my acoustic guitar, but the only place I find I'm okay is behind my father's green vinyl recliner in our den. It rests downstairs in a dark corner, and I curl fetally behind it, head between my knees, feeling as if I'm in a safe shelter—a place where I can loosen my eyes and shed some of the pain of a day.

I'm thinking about the battle ahead and I'm afraid of how this story could end. How it might be the crippling last breaths of a pneumonia-filled lung; how the virus might linger and finally take me after eating away my sight, my mind, and all my weight; how I might never win the kingdom, or marry the princess, nor be allowed to live happily ever after in my mythical world. HIV is no fantasy. And with HIV there seems to be no place for dreams.

I umbrella myself in the shadowed hue behind the recliner, my wet face hidden in the dark. Although my fear quiets, it continues so achingly in the hollow of my chest. I trace my slender fingers along the scars on my knees and think of the consequences of such a thing: my hemophilia and those necessary operations done so long ago and the factor treatments that followed. I rock on my haunches and try to summon the magical spell that will take this away, the abracadabra of another world. But it doesn't come. It grows darker, darker, darker.

Morning. Rain patters against my window, and the clouds outside cast my room in gray chalk. A slight roll of thunder shakes the rain-burdened sky, then dissipates. I lie atop my bedcovers, unmoving and listening to the thump of my family's footsteps on the floorboards above me. I shift to my side; the sheets rustle. I remain still, my eyes open but staring at nothing.

Upstairs, Mom calls out that breakfast is ready, and a few moments later Louise comes down to knock on my door.

"Mommy says it's time to eat," she relays in her thick tongue that so few of my friends can understand. She has Down syndrome and a big, pale moon-face that is her handicap's heritage. She wears thick black-rimmed glasses that enlarge her shy brown eyes, and unlike the rest of my rather slim family, her body is like a pear and she moves slow and wobbles like a penguin when she walks.

I answer that I am coming, but I lie there a few moments longer.

When I finally ascend the stairs, I see my family gathered at the table. Dad is tall and slender like a bean; his hair is thick and dark, while the decades have painted feathers of gray into the roots as well as his bushy mustache that sweeps the food and drink that passes before his lips. Mom is as an excited insect, buzzing here and there and moving so quickly that her thin outline can hardly be viewed. Her hands flutter; her feet light from spot to spot.

"Good morning," she says in a hurry from kitchen to table, bringing out a plate of scrambled eggs. She comes to me for her usual kiss, and I give her my usual cheek, and she talks on in her usual cheerful voice. "I couldn't decide on pancakes or eggs this morning, so I made both. Hope you're hungry."

I sit next to Anne. Like me, she owns the thin-bone physique of our parents. Her hair is thin and straight and hangs to the shoulders like Mom's, but is brown instead of Mom's silver-gray. She, too, has just awoken and wipes sleep from her eyes and stretches her arms in an exaggerated yawn. Then, the meal spread out and steaming before us, we eat. And later as the table is being cleared, I pour myself coffee and return again to my chair. I watch as Dad reads the paper; as Louise talks to herself and clips coupons from the newspaper sections Dad discards; as Anne leaves and returns, presenting a colorful blouse that she's considering wearing today and wishes for Mom's opinion; and as Mom declares that it will look fine and resumes sipping her own coffee across from me. Mom looks to me, smiles.

"We can get through this," she says. "We've been through a lot and we will get through this, but it'll take time. I hate to see you so down. It will get better. You have to know that. Your dad and I have already gone five years with this, and it does get better, Son."

I force a smile, but soon lose it. "How can you always be so optimistic?"

"What other way can I be?"

My best friend and I are on our way to join friends at Myrtle Beach, where we will celebrate my high-school graduation. As William drives his candy-apple Sprite convertible, he chides me on my good fortune at being long gone from a school that he has another two years to endure. The air whips around us, threatening to blow off our baseball caps. My T-shirt fills like a cotton balloon, and I feel the heaviness of salt and humidity in the air as we near the ocean. The light taste of the sea strengthens on my dry lips as we drive on. The beating sun reddens our faces and tans our arms as we yell back and forth over the drone of the European motor and American wind. It is summer, I've been on AZT for two weeks, and I've yet to disclose my HIV to anyone.

In William's car, I feel safe, timeless, untouchable like a movie star frozen on a slip of celluloid. As the sun glints off the roaring red metal, I posture the actor's part: a dashing young man happily cruising the beach highway in a catchy red convertible. I twist my shoulders, clutch the wind in my out-turned palm, and breathe out. But my HIV is still with me. Even the whip of this wind can't blow it away.

After a long silence, William questions my gloomy pall.

"Are you okay?" he asks, eyes on the road. Part Middle Eastern, part Minnesotan, William wears thin-rimmed glasses that shine brightly in the sun; the frame's right leg disappears into a mat of thick-black hair that complements a skin that easily tans.

"Yeah, of course I'm fine. Why wouldn't I be?"

He looks to me, his glasses now reflecting light so that his eyes appear as tiny suns. "Just asking."

William pulls into a gas station, parks, and starts filling up while explaining about small cars, small gas tanks, and the small islands Sprites were meant to be driven on. It is our third stop. He shakes the nozzle and bounces his car to make more room in the tank. He pays and we drive on.

The sun shines above me and the wind dries the sweat on my brow, and when I gaze into the bright sky, my eyes water. Then I start to feel those unannounced tears gathering, again, at the back of my throat. They come so often now. Roost behind my tonsils and beckon for me to let them loose. And then, I begin to cry.

"Oh my God. What's going on?"

"It's nothing. I can't talk about it." I look away and swipe my arm across my face to dab the wetness.

We arch across the Waterway bridge as boats churn summer-warmed water underneath us and as gulls canopy above. I gaze down the south channel. It disappears in the heat's haze and the curve of the horizon. Then I scan northward, following a cloud trail, catching William's eyes scrutinizing me.

"I'm scared to talk because of what you may think of me."

William assures me that what I have to say won't leave the open space of his car. I trust him, but I'm not sure what to do. But sometimes secrets come spilling out because they have to, because they must.

"I'm HIV positive."

We come to the other side of the bridge, and William drives past our Cherry Grove exit while my hands cover my rosy face. I sob again.

"Oh, man," William lets out. "Oh, man."

He says it in a whisper, barely catching in my ear over the slowing motor's idle. The wind slackens as we stall in North Myrtle Beach traffic. It is hot and getting worse. A trickle of sweat slides from beneath my armpit, runs its rivulet down my side, and disappears into my dampened clothing.

"Wow." He exhales quietly into the windshield, a long and calming breath. "Is this because of your hemophilia?"

"Yes."

My eyes close between my hands and my mind seizes upon a memory: in my parents' backyard as evening fell, Dad sipped iced tea from a sweating glass while Anne jumped rope nearby on the patio. I'd been waiting all day for the heat to abate so that I could play outside, and I'd been anxious for night, for fireflies and their light's flicker. I watched as the first tails sparked. Still able to see their bodies in the dark purple light, I chased their glimmer through the fresh-cut grass and cupped their fragile bodies in my palms, watching my hands glow a strange red as the bug's tail ignited. After I forced their flashing bodies into thick-glass Mason jars, Mom punched air holes through the lid, and when bedtime came I propped the jar on my dresser and watched their tails dance light across my room as crickets hymned songs outside my open window. Lying flat atop the sheets, catching the cool wind from an electric fan, I played like a little god and wondered if I should let these fireflies go the next day or if I should keep them here for as long as their tails still lighted, for as long as their lives still flashed. There was such power and consequence in my decision and I knew it, and I knew, too, that fate was a fragile notion.

William reaches across the seat, rests his hand on my leg. "You'll get through this," he says over the caterwaul of angry horns snarled in hot traffic. "I know it."

I tell him that I am scared, that I don't know who I should blame, that I can't understand why it happened to me, that I don't know what I am supposed to do.

"I don't know what to tell you."

"I know. There's nothing to say . . . But at least I can talk to you now."

He wheels the car past the Pavilion, turns, turns again, and we ride on the last road before ocean. The *Ripley's Believe It or Not* museum is there, advertising its miracles. Along the sidewalk, bathing suits bob and tan bodies bustle by, and I watch a group of girls pass, their strained bathing tops bouncing with their gait. One swings her blonde strands behind her shoulders and reveals to me a stretch of skin, and it doesn't seem to me that I belong anymore in such a physical world, in such a sexy place. Everyone here seems so healthy, so happy.

I wipe my eyes.

"Does anyone else know?"

"No. Well, my family. But no one else. Please keep it a secret, too. Don't tell."

"I won't. It's between us."

William's hands tightly grip the steering wheel. He stares silently ahead as we move forward slowly.

When we arrive, we find our other friends enjoying long afternoon naps and although William joins them in sleep, I am restless and in want of an ocean swim, so I head to the beach, alone.

I love this time: a warm fading sun, the constant ebb and roll of the ocean's sound, a rhythm I can count on. I remove my shoes and press my feet into the sand. The sun reddens my back as I face the sea, watching wave after wave after wave of salt water wash over a geography of silt and brine. The effortless curves of the ocean continually fold atop themselves, salty tiers of white foam. The water rides lazily around my feet, then retreats, pulling sand from underneath my soles. I wade deeper. Stroke out beyond the breakers, and from here I can see the fading blue of the horizon, the few birds that give form to this plain and shapeless sky. I slender my long body in the water and imagine the lands beyond my limited sight, cleft by the Earth's curve. I think how all that lives by water lies undetected beneath this giant flat surface.

Tucking my legs tightly to my stomach, I grab hold round the knees, dip my face in the sea, feel how the current moves me, tugs me north, then east, west, then north again in the undulating water. I'm a pale island of flesh in this quiet ocean of fish. I am moored to nothing.

Uncurling, I swim with the tide. Swim more. Toward the pier, then back. Float freely. I return to my towel on the sand, where I no longer cast a shadow. The marine sky fades black all around me while the stars begin to peek their dim faces on a moonless eve. Salt water drips from my hair, clings to my eyebrows, tightens my pores, dries to my skin. I think of nothing, but enjoy this simple moment of living. I float in it and am in no other place. And I feel inexplicably cleansed.

A MAN IN HIDING

August 1990. Although I have decided to attend college, it has crossed my mind to forgo my education and do other things: to travel while I'm still healthy, to see Rome or Venice or Paris or London or Bali or any of a host of places that one wishes to see before they die. . . . Or perhaps, instead of tiring myself out with world travel, I should do nothing other than read books at poolside and let my mind slip away from this reality. How much of my life should I change? How much should I adapt to HIV? Or perhaps, it has already been altered enough. So instead of any of these grand plans, I am here at UNC-Wilmington, or as the natives call it: UNC by the sea. I will get my college education.

My family and I hoist boxes of my belongings and cart these up two flights of stairs to my college dorm room, and after several hours the heat exhausts me. I sweat—trickles of perspiration slip from my pits. My family, too, sweats in the coastal heat, Dad the most, his cotton polo patched with dark splotches. We breathe heavy. We rest on the unmade bed. And then, feeling we've had enough recovery, Dad announces that it's time for the family to go. A mournful silence descends on us all.

"You're going to be so happy at college," Mom says with half-hearted enthusiasm. "Everything's going to work out. You'll see."

She plasters me with kisses and holds back her tears while we hug good-bye. Dad stoically hugs me—wrapping his arms around my slender frame and then, with those same long thin arms, he sweeps my family away, and they are gone. I am alone, away from home, with my HIV.

Immediately, I busy myself with unpacking. I fold my clothes in the drawers, store the snacks in the cupboard space, connect the wires for my stereo, and organize my books into milk crates—then I begin to hide my secrets: the 30cc syringes, the twenty-five gauge needles, my elastic tourniquet, my factor, and my AZT. I place my factor supplies underneath my bed and cover them with a towel. My clotting factor, however, must be refrigerated, so I wedge this behind a six-pack of Cokes, and although it can be seen, I have no other choice. I can only hope my roommate won't ask too many questions. Yet the AZT is a problem. Its discovery would ruin me. I can't keep this in the bathroom as I did at home, for I share my college bath with ten boys, any of whom could open my drawer and see the AZT bottle there, revealing immediately everything I seek to hide. I consider cloaking it underneath the bed along with the factor supplies, but the daily regime of dragging these pills out, morning and evening, would soon grow old. I rove my eyes around the room. *The closet?* No. Too accessible. *The desk?* No, though the pencil drawer has some promise. I squeeze the AZT bottle in my hands, its plastic unyielding in my tight clutch as I cast my eyes about the room for a safe hiding place. I spy my dresser, and I shove the AZT deep into a sock, it seeming safe for now.

With my things unpacked and my secrets safely hidden, I rest beside the window at my desk and arrange my reference books—dictionary, thesaurus, word menu, guide to birds in America—before settling my view on the campus yard that is now wreathed in the soft pink of an evening sunset. Tall slash pines yawn into the dusk whose horizon begins to halo with the last thin rim of daylight. Then a last ribbon of sun catches through my window and hangs in a frail quiver before the dome of night is upon me.

Before the first week of classes ends, I develop a knee bleed, another thing I must hide. "Bleed" is a hemophiliac's jargon for what doctors call a hemathrosis: the accumulation of blood in the joint. The tissue underneath my right kneecap has grown soft and spongy and the skin gives and turns pink when I press my finger to it. If students saw my swollen knee, questions would be asked, and if I answered them honestly, said I had hemophilia, well . . . connections to HIV and AIDS might be made, and I can't have that, so I must nurse myself in solitude.

Bleeds also hurt and, when in the knees, make walking difficult.

I buttress myself against the wall and various pieces of furniture as I limp gently to my door, lock it for privacy, then hobble to the refrigerator and remove my factor. Before infusing, it must come to room temperature, a process that takes about half an hour. Once, in a hurry and not letting it warm up, I infused with it fresh from the fridge, and soon I felt my heart turn into a block of ice, the freeze cooling up my vein and into the right atrium, right ventricle, left ventricle, left atrium then out, finally acclimating as it spread to my limbs and diffused with my blood. Now I know to let it warm first.

After this, I retrieve the supplies hidden underneath my bed and draw up the clear medicine into a sterile syringe and position myself under a strong light to search for a vein. Minus the sterile needles, germ-free syringes, gauze pads, and alcohol swabs, as I pump my fist and search for a vein, I feel like a junkie. Like an addict's veins, my own have become bruised and callused from constant dependence. Scarred and unreliable, they hide from my needle; collapse from overuse; blow up from too many puncture wounds; and sometimes they just leak my medicine out, which causes my skin to puff up and feel as if it is burning from the inside out.

I extend my arm, tighten the tourniquet above my elbow, pump my fist, stick the needle in my arm, and then I wait for the familiar blood return in the plastic tubing. I get a vein on my first attempt, which is not always the case. I am having a lucky day. Some days it can take three or more tries. It's on days like that when I wonder why they haven't invented a pill form of factor. At least, I say to myself, they invented a synthetically cloned product that is "safer" than the former plasma products. Then my mind imagines how, if Mononine had been invented ten years earlier, I wouldn't be HIV positive . . . but this becomes wishful and unproductive speculation.

I begin infusing, one CC at a time, so that the process takes twenty-five minutes. As I sit watching my vein; watching the needle in my arm; watching the syringe push medicine through the tubing and into my vein; and so on—there is a knock at my door. Someone calls out my name. But I remain quiet, pretend I am not here.

"I saw you go in," the voice says.

No you didn't. No you didn't.

"Hey, come on now. I just wanna borrow some paper."

Not now. Come back later.

He bangs again, rapidly, angrily. "Whatever, man. You suck. Hope you enjoy your nap." He raps heavily on the door, kicks it twice, and then is gone.

When I finish infusing, I remove the needle and place gauze over the mark left along my arm. I don't apply a Band-Aid because I've grown tired of the tediousness of always having to wear one. I discard my syringe and dirty needle in a Sharp's container, another item that has proven difficult to hide in a college dorm. It's bulky, painted red, and reads BIOHAZARD on all sides, including top and bottom. I've stored this under my bed as well, making that slip of space a veritable casket of secrets.

Now there is nothing more to do but wait for the medicine to take effect. Yet factor is not an instant cure; it takes time to work. So I fluff a pillow underneath my swollen knee, and suppress its dull throb with Tylenol, laying Vicodin at bedside in case it worsens. But I sleep. I wake in an hour and a dull fire jolts through my knee. I wince, but settle back into slumber, hoping that by morning I will be healed.

On a Sunday when the late-summer sun warms the campus, all my suitemates depart for the beach. The summer tourists have returned to their jobs, their public educations, and have left the warm ocean to us. It is like bathwater, my roommate says. He is lean like me, but older. He attended college for a while, flunked out, and is now back to give it another go. And this morning, he rose early to surf and has returned for a late breakfast, but plans to surf again. "It's too perfect. The waves. The sun. The girls. Fuck studying. You should go."

"Maybe another time. I can't today."

"What could be so important?"

I can't tell him, but today, I must drive three hours to Chapel Hill to refill my prescriptions. It is a secret mission, muling drugs from pharmacy to college dorm room. My monthly dose of AZT is almost out and I need factor, neither of which can be gotten in local pharmacies.

I fuel up and as I drive west on I-40, I notice the other cars heading east toward the shore. I spy their towels, their inflated balls, their Frisbees, and can even smell their sun-tanning lotion. I drive on, stopping for a quick lunch, and at one o'clock, after having parked in the garage and walked over the bridgeway to UNC's pharmacy located on the ground level of the main hospital, I arrive. I pull a number and wait for the pharmacist to call me. A half hour passes.

"Number 215," I hear. I rise. I go to the window.

"Yes, your name, please," the pharmacist asks, her thin glasses sliding down her thick nose.

"Shelby Smoak. I'm here to pick up my factor along with a prescription. It was phoned in earlier this week by Dr. Trum."

She types. "Oh, yes. Here it is." She leaves and then returns with the AZT, laying it on the counter while reading the computer screen. "It says here that your other prescription is in our fridge. I'll have to go get that." And she departs, but soon lobs back with a heavy paper bag that she sets beside the AZT. "There was a problem with insurance," she says casually. "They denied coverage on you, so you'll need to pay the balance and work it out with them to get reimbursed."

I breathe deeply; I don't have any money for this. But then I remember the emergency credit card Dad gave me. "Okay. I'll need to make a quick call first. How much will I owe?"

The pharmacist pushes her glasses to sit flat against her eyes as she reads from her computer screen. "Oh, honey," she says with plaintive concern, "it's almost $60,000."

"$60,000," I repeat.

"Yes . . . Your Mononine is almost $1 a unit and you need 4,000 for one treatment. And you've gotten a month's supply today. That other script ain't but about $1,000, but still. It ain't cheap. All that research and development that goes into it. That marketing too."

"And I have to pay the full amount today?"

The pharmacist fidgets with the box of factor and the small bottle of

AZT and swivels her head to peer behind me. "I wish I could help you," she says, "but yes, I'm afraid so. I can't let these go without payment."

I watch as another pharmacist in a white coat counts pills out on the table behind the lady. I see blue pills slipping into an orange-clear bottle and watch as another pharmacist begins a similar task of counting, dispensing, and labeling, repeating the process with endless precision.

"Honey," the lady before me says, drawing my attention. "You're gonna have to pay today or come back when you get it straight with insurance. I'm sure it's just some kind of silly error. But I got others I need to help, so whatcha gonna do?"

"I don't know yet. Lemme make that call and I'll be back."

"All right, chile. I'll keep this out awhile." She breaks her eyes from mine and looks over my shoulder. "Number 216."

I step aside and go in the main lobby to a row of pay phones where I dial my family collect. Mom answers and accepts the charges, and while she's excited to hear from me and launches a barrage of questions about college, my weekend, my classes, I have to quiet her and ask to speak to Dad.

"Why honey? What's wrong?"

I tell her.

"Oh my lord. That's insane. I don't know what you should do," she says. "You have to have your medicine, but oh my. That's so much money." I hear her thoughts gathering. "Hold on a minute," she says, "I'll get your father for this."

Dad answers. I hear him suck in air and guess that he's smoking as I explain the situation.

"Well, Son," he says after a pause, "there ain't any way we can pay for that today. Even if we could (and we can't) but even if we could, I don't think I'd recommend doing that. What's the odds that insurance would actually pay us back anyway? I don't trust them one lick. I couldn't take that risk." He smokes. "Goddammit," he says. "Goddammit," he says again. "That goddamn insurance is good for nothing." Smokes again. "Okay, Son, I'm gonna have to get on the horn at work tomorrow and get this thing figured out. You got enough factor for another day or two?"

"Yes. I should be okay. I have two treatments left."

"How 'bout the other?"

I pause. "I'm gonna be out tonight."

"Tonight! Goddammit, Son. Goddammit, goddammit." He smokes. "You gotta refill your medicine before you get that low. Damn." He puffs again. "Okay. Nothing to do about it now. That's the one for a thousand?"

"Yes, Dad. That's what she said."

"All right then. Reckon you can put that on the card and hope to hell we get reimbursed. Goddamn, Son. Damn." I hear the lighter flicking in the phone line. Then a long puff. "Okay. The other you're gonna have to leave. But once it's straight, and I hope it's straight before the sun goes down tomorrow, but once it is straight, I'm afraid you're gonna have to turn around and drive back for it."

I'm thinking about classes and homework and the fatigue of driving there and back again, but really what choice do I have? This is important. This is real life.

"Okay. I'll do it. I don't guess there's any other choice."

"I reckon not and I'm sorry for it, Son. Awful sorry. But these things happen. Hope you understand. There's just no way for us to pay this thing outright. It's too much goddamn money. Especially when you've got insurance!"

I hang up and return to the pharmacy window and hand over the Visa for the AZT which, once accepted, I slip into my backpack, leaving the factor.

Monday afternoon, Dad calls.

"It's figured out," he says. "I got it all straight now, Son. Some damn notion they had that we'd dropped you at eighteen. Goddamn them. Think they must do that to all their high-profile clients. Anyway, called the pharmacy and you're good to go. It's there and ready for you. You can pick it up anytime but remember that hospital pharmacy closes at five."

"Okay. Thanks, Dad. I'll go tomorrow. I'll have to miss my afternoon class, but it's the only time I can go."

And when we hang up, I crack open my philosophy textbook and read ahead for the lecture I will have to miss.

THE REGULAR

December 1990. It is a familiar scene: the hospital examination room. Here, I wait for Dr. Trum and my six-month checkup, which I have fit in over the holiday break. I twirl my fingers round, lean my head against the wall, and pretend to sleep, but can't, so I read posters on the wall—one a diagram of the HIV virus. *So that's inside me,* I think as I study the blue cell and those broad red arrows that mark HIV's path of invasion. It is as a military map: the Visigoths crossing the Danube, the Germans the English Channel. The invading medicine sallies against HIV from the left, the right, above, and below, and, as the graph depicts it, AZT vanquishes HIV. I cross my fingers and hope it so. It has now been six months since I have been on AZT and today's test results should indicate the drug's success, or lack of.

The door opens; the dentist enters. She looks into my mouth, peels my lips up and down to reveal my gumline, and she picks her metal instrument into my molars.

"It's soft back there. I'm afraid you may be developing a cavity which we need to take care of. Can you come in to have it done?"

"A filling?"

"Yes. You'll need to factor, of course, before the procedure."

She offers me a Monday in late January.

"What about a Tuesday or Thursday? I'll have to miss my Monday classes next semester, and I'd rather not."

The dentist consults her calendar, leaves to make a phone call, and returns with an available Thursday in February. I accept. Then a half hour passes before the physical therapist enters, waking me from a light doze.

"I'm not sure I need to see you today. I'm seeing the orthopedist in the afternoon."

"Are you? That's good. But all my measurements are routine. I visit all the hemophiliacs in the clinic. It's my job." She lays her folder atop the desk to indicate that she's staying. "It won't take long. I promise." She bends me, stretches me, extends me, measures me, and finally leaves me, a little more exhausted.

Next, the social worker.

"So how are you?" she asks.

"Fine." I trace my finger along the white paper covering the examination table.

"Okay. That's good." She writes some notes down. "Now, do you care to be more specific?"

I feel she's pressing for some confession, something about the unbearable weight of HIV, but what can she really do for me? What will I get from crying my infected heart out to her? "Okay . . . Well . . . I like school, college."

"Now where are you? UNCW, right?"

"Yes."

"And have you felt adjusted there?"

"Yes. Sure. It's fine. Like I said."

She scribbles on her yellow memo pad, pauses, and looks at me with dark eyes that catch a flicker of sunlight from the window.

"And what about your HIV? How does that make you feel?"

Like a victim. Like a man before the firing squad.

"I can't imagine what that has done to you," she says. "But you've got to know that you are not alone."

Yes I am.

"We have groups here at the hospital that meet and help one another cope with this, and there are hemophiliacs just like you who come. Perhaps it would do you some good to talk about this with one of them. Have you talked to your family at all?"

No. Not really.

"What about a friend?" she continues. "I know it must be hard to open up, especially with the stigma attached to HIV, but do you have a friend that you've told?"

I stay silent. I have nothing to say.

She purses her lips, retrieves a card from her pocket, and passes it to me. "Here's this if you change your mind and decide to come to a meeting. We have different ones, and I'm sure we could accommodate your schedule. We even have some that meet on Saturdays. I can't make you come, but I do think it would help. You have a right to be upset, and this could be a forum for working through that. You shouldn't go this alone. It's too much for anybody and there are lots of people willing to help."

After the social worker leaves, I stretch out on the table and roll onto my side and gaze out the window to the parking lot below. From here, the cars remind me of the Matchbox toys I once played with. Then there was such simple joy in pushing a metal car across a linoleum floor or atop a bedspread or through a carpet of shag—just going from one side to another without a concern of why or what for.

Overhead, the sun radiates feebly through the winter sky. A sphere of weak fire in a dome of cold blue, it hangs pendulant in an endless ceiling of pewter.

Eventually, Dr. Trum enters. We shake hands and then assume our roles: he the doctor, me his patient.

"It's probably been a strange couple of months for you since we last met," he says as a way of transition. "So, how have you been anyway?"

"Okay, I guess."

He shines a light in my eyes to check my pupils. He lays a cold stethoscope against my chest to listen to my still-beating heart, my breathing lungs.

"Sounds good here." He removes his stethoscope and drapes it across his neck. He examines the scars on my knees. He presses softly with his thumb and index finger against the swelling in my ankles, both tender with blood.

"You've had a few bleeds in these, I see. Probably due to all the walking you're doing on campus."

"Yes. Nothing major, but kept me down for a day or two."

"That's good. Just remember that rest is best when these things happen . . . I see that you're visiting the orthopedist today," he says as he flexes my ankles and measures their inability to bend. "He may recommend a walking aid for you. Something to reduce your bleeding into these joints. My worry is about your increased bleed episodes since starting college. I fear arthritis may soon set in. We want to slow that down as much as possible." He sits down and opens my folder, the size of an "S" encyclopedia.

"Are you tolerating the AZT? Had any side effects? Dizziness? Nausea? Light-headed? Muscle spasms?"

"No."

"Good. That's good. We want this stuff to work for you." He jots notes. "Have you skipped any doses?"

"No. Well . . . Once I forgot to take it before bedtime. But that's only once."

"Hmmm . . . Well, okay. But you can't make a habit of that. You have to stay on top of HIV with the AZT," he says to me with a fixed and intent stare. "Don't skip any doses," he adds before turning his attention to a slip of paper. "I have your lab numbers back from last visit, and unfortunately your CD-4 counts are still dropping."

I inhale quietly and feel sorrow drawing down my heart.

"We're going to keep you on AZT. But soon, not today, but soon we need to think about adding some preventive measures with AZT. We want to stop the infections before they start and try to halt them before they spread. The thing you need to keep in mind, though, is that we are still learning about this thing. That things are changing every day with HIV, and that it is going to get better. I've got patients with counts a lot lower than yours and they're doing great, leading successful lives. We're finding that this thing just might be manageable," he says as he closes my folder and rises to leave.

Ending there, he shakes my hand and pats me on the back as a father might. As if that's enough.

Next, I follow the familiar hallways to the orthopedic clinic, stopping at the snack bar along the way for a quick lunch. While Dr. Trum treats my hemophilia (and now my HIV), the orthopedist repairs the damage internal bleeding enacts upon my body, for factor isn't enough to heal me. I am a regular here too. The receptionist knows my smile, the nurse my weight and temperature, the doctor my scars and deformed bones.

The summer I was eight I had a synovectomy. I spent June in traction, July in water tanks, and August and September on crutches relearning how to walk. By October, I could hobble about the schoolyard, happy, I suppose, to be walking again. And then when I was ten, the orthopedist had to cut me again to drain pooled blood from my knee. Seven weeks later—after traction and therapy—I was discharged to limp about on crutches until my legs could hold my body again, which happened two months later. Those surgeries' memories, however, are the long red scars forever etched along the uneven curve of my patella. Due to their unsightliness, I seldom wear shorts, and then only to swim.

In the orthopedist's waiting room, I rustle through a magazine as the dull afternoon passes. A young girl, a white cast sealed round her leg, crutches to a nearby chair, where she lowers herself with her mother's aid; a man across from me lifts a soda with his good arm, the other braced in a sling; and a boy wheels across the waiting room, his legs lifeless and dangling below him and his chair.

My name is called. I rise. I greet the nurse and am told to visit X-ray. The doctor has ordered a series of photographs.

There, I disrobe. Goosebumps rise along my flesh, and I retrieve a thin white blanket, wearing it like a toga, while I wait again in a smaller, more secluded alcove. When the technician enters, he explains that I am to have a full workup today, that all my joints are going to be X-rayed.

"And how long will that take?"

"Hopefully, if they all come out, I can have you out of here in an hour."

He lays me on the metal table, slips a film tray into his machine, aims the camera's lens over my knee, disappears behind a steel shield, and snaps a button. I hear a click; then he returns, stretches my legs out, pushes my arms over my head, and positions the X-ray, an act he assumes with tedious exactness and with no sense of time nor of my discomfort before he darts behind his screen again. The machine clicks again, and again he returns to pull my body as if it is taffy.

As he repeats the process, again and again, the cold slab of metal chills my skin. He X-rays my knees, my ankles, my hips, my elbows, my wrists, and my spread fingers, and when, two hours later, I am given the large red folder containing these pictures, I pass this to the orthopedic nurse, who promptly thanks me and tells me to wait again, adding that the doctor will see me momentarily. I sit. The girl with the cast and the man with the sling are gone, but the boy now sleeps with his chair parked against the waiting room wall. My head feels light, my stomach empty, and I curse myself for not stopping for something to eat after the X-ray. It is now well into the afternoon, and my lunch isn't holding me. I should have been more prepared and brought something: a granola bar, a pack of crackers, a juicy steak.

When the orthopedist and his resident—a foreign medical student with oil-black hair, dark eyebrows, and a thick accent—arrive in the room where I wait, storm clouds gather in the dark sky, casting an ominous glow on the late day. I am again pulled and twisted, bent and straightened, measured and assessed. The orthopedist requests that I walk down the clinic hallway, so I remove my shoes and socks, roll up my jeans, and walk as best I can. A nurse hurries by with her quick and easy step, and the steady patter of her soft white shoes echoes through the corridor. My body gives on my left side, and my knees do not straighten as they should, but I walk (limp), turn around (yaw like a ship), walk (limp) more.

"Okay. That's good enough," the orthopedist calls out.

When we return to the room, he clips a few of my X-rays to the light-board and places a thoughtful finger to his bottom lip. His eyes have a faraway gaze and are deep in study.

"It looks as if you've suffered more damage to your knees and ankles, and you're losing rotation in your left hip." The medical student takes notes. "I suspect this is due to several things. For one, you have hemophilia and this is its nature. For another, you are now at college and, well, you're probably walking more than you used to. This increased activity is probably adding further aggravation to your joints, which are already under strain from hemophilia. This isn't an ideal situation and we have to consider ways to counteract this deterioration of your joints." He again places his finger to his lips, removes it. "A cane could help relieve some of the stress you're experiencing, especially on your left side, which seems to be deteriorating more rapidly."

"A cane?"

"Yes. A cane."

"But I'm only eighteen. Nobody has a cane at eighteen."

"I understand the stigma, but you're different. You know that. And you're now walking with a noticeable limp. We don't want your gait to worsen too quickly." He gathers my X-rays and returns them to his folder. "As for the cane, you don't have to use one, of course. I only think it could help. You've had an increase of bleeding episodes this fall, and I think you need to consider ways to reduce those. Each one does more and more damage to your joints, and if too much damage occurs . . . well . . . we'll have to consider other methods for treatment."

I understand his meaning here, and I'm certainly not wishing for another operation. Not now. Not ever again.

"Think on it," he says, shaking my hand on his way to another patient.

Outside, a storm begins. The wind chafes my cheeks as I walk to the parking lot, so I tighten my scarf around my neck, it binding round me like a noose. The sky—heavy and pregnant with winter—begins to sift freezing rain upon me.

On the highway to my parents', as the cars edge forward with caution, the sleet pings on my windshield and gathers in the corners as grains of translucent white. It salts the grass and tar-black roadside while the trees—having become hazy and borderless—are washed flat against a gray sky. I grip the steering column and climb the Piedmont hills with care.

Going home for Christmas, I drive slowly. The snow-ice dusts the roadways, and the salt trucks I pass are too few to keep the highways clear. On the bridge that spans the Yadkin River, my lightweight truck loses purchase. I tense and place a firm grip on the steering column as I slip up the bridge—an arabesque of ice and snow stretched over a river, blue and stiff with cold.

Turning onto my parents' street, the snow thickens. Patches like thrown flour splotch my windshield, and when I finally pull into the driveway, the yard is speckled in white, and a long, green-white lawn follows the right side of the house and dips into the backyard before finally being halted from unrolling any further by the rusted barbed-wire fence. It looks like a rolling gumdrop dusted with powdered sugar. I am relieved to be here safe.

Mom rushes out, coatless. Without a way to call her and let her know I was safe, she has worried.

"Oh, we're so glad to see you," she says, hurrying to me. "Dad and I have been worried sick about you driving in this awful weather. They're saying that the roads are icing over and it's already sleeting. Is it as bad as they say?"

"It's pretty bad. I wouldn't suggest going anywhere tonight."

"Well, we're not. Everybody's here. We're just waiting on you." She pulls me to her and hugs me. "We're just glad you're here safe. How did it go today in Chapel Hill?" I pass her my duffel bag full of dirty laundry. "What did the doctor say?" The snow whirls around us, peppers our hair.

"They said I'd live forever." I smile to her as I hoist my backpack across my shoulders and gather CDs in my hands.

"Oh, that's not funny, Son. You shouldn't joke like that."

"They said you and Dad should get me a cane for Christmas."

"A cane?" Mom scrunches her face with worry. "Well, your father and I had concerns when we saw the size of that campus, but a cane? Does the doctor really think it's that necessary? Would you have to always use it?"

"I don't know. Guess so."

We both grow quiet, the snow continuing around us.

"Well, come in. We're so glad you're finally home for a few days. We've hardly gotten to see you this fall."

Inside, Mom has the table set for supper and the house decorated for the holidays. Nutcrackers stand in all the corners, garland twirls along the banister, and Christmas candles adorn the piano and the furniture, and when I take my bags downstairs to my room, the den smells sweetly of pine and the tree shimmers with silver and gold ornaments.

"Your dad and I just got that up last weekend," Mom says when I stop to look. "It was different not having you to help this year." She walks to the tree, reaches for a fallen ornament resting on the skirt. "Look here." She cups it in her hand. "Do you remember when you made this?"

I look to the ceramic star painted by an inexpert hand, and admit that I don't remember making it.

"First grade. We had that house in Indiana and you had just started at the elementary school there, and that year Louise lost her shoe in the snow and it wasn't until spring that your dad found it laying over by the bird bath." She stretches to replace the ornament on a green branch of spruce. "This is what you gave us that year."

"Well, I didn't make any of those in college, so it's good you kept it."

"Ha-ha."

In my room, I unpack my things and then reach for a book to read. I prop my feet on my bed, turn to the first page. But it is not long before Louise comes down to tell me it's time to eat, so I mark my place and go to join my family at the holiday table.

We all look out the window beside the dining room table and watch the snow still being drawn down in a slow drift of white.

"Maybe this year we'll have a white Christmas," Mom says.

"Maybe," Dad says, pulling his napkin up to wipe his mustache. "Stranger things have happened."

"I'd love a white Christmas. That would be perfect," Anne says as she, too, gazes out to the snow piling in our yard.

ANA

January 1991. Ana was my first, my only. It happened in a musky garage where beetles scuttled across concrete walls to tango with the cobwebs, where musical instruments lay strewn and disregarded, where dust motes floated in the phantom evening light from outside. My high school friends and the band we jammed in long since retired for the night, Ana and I reclined on a mattress, on a sultry night in June—my birthday.

"Are you ready?" she whispered, coiling her shaven leg around mine, knowing this was my first time.

I unrolled the condom just as my more experienced friend had shown me. "I'm ready."

I kissed her. We pressed our bodies together. I was in. I was out. I was done.

Afterwards, Ana and I sprawled in the lavender twilight, whispered endearing words of foreverness, and snugged our naked bodies against each other. I knew nothing of love, and yet I said I did as I held her tightly. We kissed more. We played our hands together, and we began again. And I had no idea then of our danger.

These thoughts return to me as I again read the Christmas card Ana has mailed. It says she thinks about me often, and naturally, I think of her, feeling an inordinate responsibility to her. Dr. Trum had asked about my sexual relations, but I assured him that I had retained my virginity all my high school years. I was the minority statistic, I had quipped. And he did not press me, but asked that I be forthcoming when I began having sex. Often, I have thought of Ana and have retraced our actions, scrutinizing them for any slip—a split condom perhaps, or a time we pressed forward without protection, but I can recall none. It seems our fear of pregnancy kept us safe from so much other than that.

Yet still, I must confide in Ana and warn her that our *le sport* was not as carefree as we thought. But how can a man as young as me be expected to have a conversation such as this? How can any man?

When I return to campus after winter break, I call her. I will be as an old boyfriend calling his once-girlfriend, I say to myself as the phone rings.

Ana sounds excited and says she is glad to hear from me, and soon we fall into a lengthy conversation about our lives since we parted. I am swept away by her easy laughter and her voice's soft cadence. I can't remember why we broke up. One year, we were high school juniors dating, having sex; then we were seniors parting for separate colleges, and ending the relationship seemed the thing to do.

"Why don't you visit sometime?" Ana asks during a pause.

"Okay. When's a good time?"

"How about next weekend? My roommate's out of town."

"Okay. Next weekend."

And when we hang up, I feel happier than I've felt in months. My body is warm. My breath easy. Yet HIV is there to remind me of sadness. I bury it. For now.

When Friday comes, I speed along Interstate 40, closing the distance between Wilmington and Greensboro, Ana and me. I'm so excited to see her that I arrive almost an hour early and kill the extra time by napping in my cab as twilight becomes night, but yet my stomach roils when I think of HIV.

Later, from the dorm's front desk, the R.A. pages Ana, who soon skips down the hallway and rushes me with a hug. Her hair tickles my chin and smells like fresh spring flowers. She presses her pink and full cheeks again my slender neck, and she holds me with arms that are warm and nourishing like freshly baked bread. Ana says she can't believe I came, squeezes me, says again how she can't believe I came and tells me how good it is to see me.

She rushes off to her room to gather her things and then we eat out at a Mexican restaurant, talking and laughing like old times. And after dinner, we stroll the campus, hold hands beneath the southern stars, and kiss beside a Jeffersonian column as the blush of winter rubs deep roses into our cheeks. We easily fall into our old roles—she my girlfriend, I her boyfriend. It is as it was before. We kiss and hold one another as if this is the only thing to do in the world.

When we return to her dorm, she distracts the night-watch while I tiptoe past to her room, my bag in hand, slipping in undetected. Ana follows and shuts the door behind us.

"I missed you," she says clasping my hands, touching my lips with hers.

"I missed you, too."

She removes her shirt. I mine. And we move to her bed.

"I don't want to go too far tonight," she says.

"Me, either."

So, we tease one another's desire with our hands, our mouths, our burning breath. Ana leans over me and covers me under her sheet. She runs her hands across my bare chest, my skinny legs, my strong spirit. We indulge in the petting of young lovers.

"Oh, we have to stop," Ana says, retracting. "This is going too far."

She pushes away from me, letting out a rush of air as she falls into the mattress. Our breathing calms and my drumming heart quiets.

"I'm so glad you came to see me," Ana says, playing her hands along my thin bone. "I was hoping you'd call if I sent that card. I wasn't sure how else to get your attention." She wets her lips and gingerly kisses me before pulling away with a strange look on her face. "Shelby," she says, changing her tone. "I think you're bleeding."

Startled and embarrassed, I check myself in Ana's mirror and see that I have a bleeding razor cut.

"Dammit," I say. "You did this . . . All that wrestling underneath the covers has done this." I press a Kleenex to the cut.

"Looks like a shaving accident to me. But I'll take part of the blame. Do you want a Band-Aid?"

"Yes. I don't want to bleed on your pillow."

She rises from her bed, goes to a small box above her sink and then comes toward me with the Band-Aid. "Here. Let me put that on for you."

I freeze. Think of my blood, of HIV.

"No. I can do it. I need to take care of my own problems. I'm a big college boy, now. I need to do this myself."

"Fine. But I'm buying you an electric razor."

Ana relinquishes the Band-Aid, which I secure over the cut; then I slip back into bed where Ana nuzzles against me.

"It's nice to not be lonely anymore," she whispers into the night as we fall asleep.

Another weekend as I drive to see Ana, my truck's odometer measures the real distance of our love. I crack my window and the breeze chills me while the wind drones out the Stone Roses album straining from my tiny dashboard speakers. The asphalt clips underneath my tires, and the city lights dance neon rainbows as I streak through winter twilight.

When I arrive, Ana's dorm is quiet. The thrall and hum of young scholars has been replaced by the hollow echo of a few pattering steps and the distant sound of faceless voices.

I call Ana's name down the hallway toward her room. She soon answers back.

"It's so quiet here," I tell her when she greets me.

"They've all left for some party. My roommate, also, has left for the night. We'll be all alone."

I smile. Ana smiles back.

We go to a movie; then we return to her silent dorm, slinking down the vacant hallway in the giddy embrace of young lovers. Ana playfully kicks open her door and flips on a lamp in the corner that casts her room in a romantic glow. She stands by her bedside, rubs her hand across its coverlet.

"What should we do now?" she asks. My skin prickles. My heart flutters.

"What should we do?" I repeat, playing the game Ana has begun. And yet, my mind is nettled by HIV. But I suppress it.

She pulls me to her, pushes her warm hands underneath my shirt and sweater, and strokes my chest. She lures me to her bed, where I begin fumbling with her blouse. And when she climbs on top of me, her long hair catches in my mouth, and I lift my hand to hook her dangling strands behind her ear; then I breathe into her ear and kiss her neck. She sighs with pleasure, her hands struggle with my jeans' zipper.

"Wait," I say.

"We have waited."

She moves lower. Then, she is breathing on me. I can't look at her, so I stare at the ceiling, studying leak stains that spread out like continental maps. I swell. Ana stops and pulls herself to my lips where we heave and grope and grind our hips together, the thin fabric between us our only restraint.

"I have condoms underneath my bed," Ana whispers into my ear.

My mind tugs at me, but when Ana unrolls a condom along me, I let her. We become two bodies, one movement, and we press our desire as far as it will go.

When the moment ends, Ana fills a glass of water at her sink, drinks deeply, and then offers it to me. I swallow, pause for a breath of air, and finish it off. It is cool and tastes like nothing, but is everything. Ana rests the glass on her floor and returns to bed where I slip an arm around her.

In the corner, the lamp burns, dimly, moodily. Ana rises up to kiss me, and she then shifts to fit in the slip of space between my arm and my heart. Her eyes close, open, close, and then close.

I'm thinking of how to tell her about my HIV . . . but I am asleep.

Later, I awaken and get up to turn out the lamp and refill the water glass. I sip while standing over Ana and watching her sleep in the gray moonlight. Curled onto her side, the sheet tucked to her neck, and with strands of her blonde hair splayed out onto the pillow, she breathes in such gentle and easy peace. I take a few more sips before slipping back into her arms.

When morning comes, we drive into the country. Despite it being cold, it is a lovely day: the sun is out, the sky is clear, and a car ride seems fun. We don't speak of last night, but I can't loosen it from my mind. I'm restless and need to confess. Yet I don't know what to say, for HIV does not enter our conversation.

She leans against me and tells me she is happy.

"Are you happy to be with me again?" she asks.

"I am."

We drive into winter. The trees are bare and the meadows we pass are humped with the heaviness of rolled hay, and the geese file over us as we pass the withered barnlots of a past life. Ana stretches out her tender hand, and I grip it as I steer to nowhere in particular.

Ana visits me in Wilmington. She has told me to be waiting, so I wait, realizing that I have to tell her. It has gone too far.

Ana knocks at my door. I inhale deeply and then I let her in.

"Oh, it's been too long," she says, placing her bag at the foot of my bed. She then draws me on top of her and my bed. "I've missed you." And we're at each others' clothes, manipulating clasps, navigating fabric.

"Wait. We have to talk."

Ana freezes. "Talk?" Her face looks troubled.

"It's not what you think."

"How do you know what I think?"

"I can see it in your eyes. This isn't a breakup talk. This is harder to say."

I lie down beside her, stare at my ceiling—a wilderness of white.

"Well, what is it?" Ana trifles her fingers along a dangling sweater string, coils it tightly around her index joint. "You have to tell me now."

"You know I have hemophilia?" She nods yes. "Well, when I was a little boy, something happened to me."

"Is this about your operations?"

"Sort of."

"Well, I just wanted you to know that your scars don't bother me."

"It's not that. It's about some blood I received through a transfusion."

Ana pauses, her mind sifting for meaning. "Oh, no," she exhales. "Oh, no," she repeats. Her eyes water. "You?" she asks softly. She wipes away a tear. "You?"

"Yes, me."

She buries her face into my chest while her body shakes against my heart. My arms enwrap her, my face looks skyward, and I cry, too. I flashback to those nights with Ana: our naked bodies, the bitter scent of passion.

"How long have you known?" she asks after a long and labored lull.

"They told me when I turned eighteen. After I graduated high school."

Ana sobers. She dabs her tears with a Kleenex drawn from my bedside dispenser. "Were we . . . ?"

"Safe?"

"Were we?"

"Yes. We were safe. We always used condoms."

Ana straightens herself in my bed, leans against the headboard, and looks out the window. She wipes a pale hand across her wet eyes. I gaze past her.

"So, we've been safe? Just tell me that what we do is safe. Just tell me that."

"Yes, Ana. It is safe."

She draws herself to me, stares at me with red eyes. She straddles me and yanks off her shirt, revealing the tiny birthmark above her navel. Then she pushes her shirt up to her stomach and frees her pink panties where I can feel the press of her wetness on me.

"What are you doing?" I ask as she unclasps my belt.

"Well . . . I can't be in a relationship without sex. Not now. Not with you."

"Are you sure?"

She kisses me. "Yes. I'm sure."

We say nothing, but lock hands and squeeze one another and reach for protection when we are ready. And later, when I trace my finger along the curve of Ana's arm, which rests outside the sheets, she breathes quiet in the afternoon while my own mind labors over the burden of HIV.

Outside, a steady rain drizzles on the coastal pines, wetting the rusted needles that litter the winter courtyard. The constant patter of rain reverberates off the roof, the window, the sidewalk. There is nothing but this sound, stillness and quiet.

The next weekend when I visit Ana, we have sex and sleep and have more sex, only breaking apart to eat, to shower, or to shift ourselves after sex. We press our bodies together to assure we are real. Ana explains how HIV has brought us closer, how it has given everything urgent clarity.

"Now I love you even more," she declares.

April. Having spent Easter with our families and now, the holiday ended, we say goodbye before heading back to school. Wrapped around one another on her parents' couch, Ana and I press together and then catch our breath while the television flickers blue light over our skin.

"I'm going to miss you," Ana says, turning to face me. "I can't wait until summer. Then we'll see each other every day." She hugs me tightly and rubs her bare ankle along my calf and settles her face to my quiet heart. I hold her loosely and trace the notches of her spine. "I feel your heart beating," she says. "It's really fast."

"We did just have sex."

"I know, but it's really loud and fast."

She continues to listen, and then I feel a tear against me.

"You okay baby? What's wrong?"

Ana wipes her eyes. "I worry about you. What if you get sick? What are we to do then?"

Ana's question hangs in the dark gulf between us. "What if . . . ," I say, trailing off.

She breaks my hold of her so our noses touch, and I can see the sorrow her eyes veil.

"It's not like it'll happen right away. It takes time."

"But what if you start? What if you get your first infection?"

"Then I'll deal with it. I can't live constantly imagining how I might die."

"I know that, but what about us?" Ana plays our fingers together and makes a steeple of them. "If you get sick, you have to promise me something."

"Promise you?"

"Yes."

"I can't promise till I know what it is."

"Just promise, okay. For me." She places her palm on my face. A tear slides the short line of her nose. "Promise me that if you start getting sick that you'll marry me. You will marry me won't you?"

"Is that what you want, Ana? To marry someone who will likely leave you a young widow?"

"No, I don't want that to happen. But if it does, I want to have something of yours to carry on. I want to have your name. Promise me that. Say it for me."

"Okay. I promise that if I get sick I'll marry you."

She throws her arms around me and cries into my chest. "I love you so much," she says. "I love you so much, I love you so much," she repeats as an unending chant.

When Ana quiets, we remain gripped to one another in silence. The television bounces light through the room and gives us laughter where there is none. Then we fall into a light sleep and let it renew our troubled hearts as much as it can.

When I awaken, I have no sense of the time, but can feel that it's late, so I nudge Ana.

"I have to go. It's getting late."

"No," she says sleepily. "Not yet. Just a few more minutes." She curls herself into a ball next to me, tightens her arms around me. I lie against her and watch as her mother's cat grooms itself underneath the hazy lamp light. The cat methodically licks a paw and swipes it across an ear, repeating this movement several times before settling its head against the carpet.

"Ana . . . Ana, I have to go. It's a long drive to Wilmington."

"I know." She rises and drapes a coverlet over her while I dress. "I'll show you out."

Over the threshold of her open door, we hug goodnight while a moth flutters near our kissing faces and then disappears inside her house.

"See you in a few weekends?" she asks.

"Yes, two weeks."

"That seems like forever right now."

"It'll pass and soon we'll have the whole summer together."

"Yes. That's something to look forward to."

I wave one last time from my truck's cab and Ana waves back, wiping her tears with her other hand. Then the night tents around me. The brilliant stars scatter themselves across a dark canvas while the faint scent of dogwood drifts through my cab and is then gone. And when I think of Ana and of marriage, fear envelops me. *Would we be happy? Would I?* My stomach twists with the thought of such a sad matrimony.

SANDWICH INTERLUDE

SUMMER 1991. ANA AND I SPRAWL ONTO ONE OF OUR PARENTS' couches every evening and, when we are alone, we shed our clothes and press our desire until we are shaking with pleasure. Then we settle into familiar spoons and twirl fingers in the dark.

"Oh, I'm going to hate when summer ends," she says. "It's so great having you here every day. It's spoiling me."

"Me, too."

We kiss and kiss and Ana slips her hand to my hips to see if I'm ready again.

During the day, however, I work at a sub shop. I earn minimum wage and am congratulated on my hard work and dependability by my manager. And while the job gives me money for gas, dinner dates, movies, and CDs—after work, my legs ache, my ankles swell like oranges, and my knee joints crackle like puffed rice. Tonight, I can hardly walk, so I lumber to the refrigerator for my factor. I take it out, treat, and fall asleep, exhausted and hurting, only waking when Ana calls to come over.

Through the June heat and into July, I sweat over the steak grill, and every few days, my ankle flares up, and I must treat. Tonight, my ankle pounds pain, and I'm limping severely as I slice ham, grill steak, and heat meatballs. Hopeful that I can leave when we close at eleven, I start the cleaning list:

Take apart meat slicer and wipe; Windex display case; store extra meat, lettuce, tomatoes, onions, and cheese in freezer; scrape grill; clean countertops;
scrub toilets; mop floor; take out trash. And at 10:50 as I heft the last bag of
garbage into the dumpster, a Caravan cruiser circles into the empty parking
lot and a six-member family unloads and lobs toward the restaurant. If I let
them in, I'll have to reclean everything, and it'll be another hour before I
can clock out, so I act quickly: I rush the door with the keys, secure the lock,
and scurry away to cower behind the counter. A man yanks on the door. Then
again, louder and with more force. My heart palpitates. He pounds the glass.

"I know you're still fucking in there," he huffs. "You ain't supposed to be
goddamn closed. Your sign ain't even off."

His anger echoes throughout the sub shop while I massage my swollen
ankle, praying for him to leave.

"Goddamn, you. Goddammit." He pounds again, beating the glass front
in rapid-fire succession with the neon OPEN sign flashing beside him. Hairs
lift along my arms. I pull my legs to my chest and pray again for him to
leave. Then I hear the scruff of retreat, doors slamming, a vehicle coughing
to life, and the skid of tires pealing off.

I count to twenty and, feeling safe, ease my head above the countertop.
The parking lot glows from the streetlights and, save that weak yellow light,
is black and empty. I slowly rise and, scanning the lot to reassure myself he's
gone, I scurry to unplug the OPEN sign, noticing then the smear of hand-
prints and boot-marks on the glass; so I fetch the cleaner and hastily scrub
away these marks before locking up and limping to my truck.

At home I infuse and then comfort my ankle atop a pillow and gently
rest it against an ice pack. I lie back on my mattress and exhale deeply.
Upstairs, Mom calls down.

"Your dad and I are going to bed," she says. "What time do you work
tomorrow?"

"Early. I have to leave at ten."

Then the house quiets. The night chirps, and I drift off.

The next morning, I wrap my ankle in an Ace bandage, and I fit on my shoe as
best I can. I swallow several Tylenol and pocket a handful more. Then I leave.

When lunchtime arrives, the Caravan returns and my heart seizes with panic. In overalls splattered with white paint, the man saunters in and motions to my manager, and they talk. The man smiles a large mouth of yellow teeth when I am told to make him a free meatball sub. I return his smile, but neither of us speaks. When he finishes eating, he balls up the wrapper and tosses it toward the trash, missing the hole and spilling food.

"Oops," he says. "Guess you'll have to clean that up." Then he leaves.

After lunch, my boss corners me around a boxed fortress of sub rolls and tells me I won't get my monthly raise and that, additionally, he's knocking my pay down by ten cents an hour. He debases my qualities as an employee, and I lowly hang my head, offering my subservience.

Angry, I huff outside and slump against the stairwell. The hot air chokes me and sears my lungs. Sweat beads on my forehead and dampens my work shirt. Leaning across the railing, I think of what to do and decide that I should quit. The job is wearing me down and I need to heal.

So I limp inside, and I find my boss at his desk, leaned back with his feet propped up.

"I'd like to put in my two-week notice," I say.

He glances up. "No. Don't bother. You can quit now."

"Okay. I quit then. And here's the shirt for your next employee," I say, tearing off the shirt and throwing it at him.

He jolts up and aims his finger at me. "Don't ever ask me for a recommendation! You won't get it from me!"

"Fine!"

"I mean it. Ever!"

"Fine!"

When I leave, he slams the door and my restaurant career ends forever.

COLLEGE

September 1991. Ana and I have been seeing each other every other weekend since school resumed, but that's getting harder to manage. I'm busy; my workload has increased threefold; consequently, I'm in the library every evening and now need the weekends for study.

Tonight, I recline in my favorite chair—the one tucked against the large window that stares out upon the campus walk—and my heavy bookbag rests at my feet, yet instead of reading my coursework, I thumb another medical journal in the hope of understanding more about me. In college I've learned about research, about finding answers to things you don't understand. But today the news isn't promising. Long-term studies of AZT indicate that side effects such as nausea and muscle contractions develop, or worse, that HIV becomes resistant to AZT.

I let the journal slip into my lap while my gaze drifts outside to the longleaf pines blowing in the campus breeze. I think of a night not long ago when I awoke with a muscle spasm in my calf, another when my foot curled itself inside my shoe and required coaxing to return to normal. And then there is my nausea. Sometimes in the early morning as I eat breakfast, or later in the evening during dinner, it comes. I ignore it, blame it on a steady diet of coffee, and cure it with slow steady breathing or perhaps by lying down, or if nothing else works, I rush to the closest toilet and unload my insides. I have thought that HIV caused this, but now I wonder if it's AZT. And if so, what can I do? It seems I am moored to illness. My stomach sinks.

In my chair as the sun descends behind the campus lawn, I recline in the casual pose of a college student caught up in deep thought. I have now carried the knowledge of my HIV for a year. My only confessions have been to William and to Ana. Still, I hide it. And I suppose, too, that I am still dying, a thought too difficult to conceptualize with any honest attachment.

Here I've stumbled too close to reality, and I must let it out. This is not uncommon. Tears spill forth in the quiet of an untraveled book row, or in the morning shower, or in the cotton sheets I sleep beneath. And when I've folded my torn heart over and wrung it dry of ache, when I've embraced mortality and squeezed it hatefully and lovingly and hatefully again, I must then move on.

October 1991. Friends persuade me to join the crew team as a coxswain, and today is my first morning of practice. As I wait in front of my suite for my roommate to return with his car, the cold bites at my gloved hands, so I cup them to my mouth and breathe heat into them. Last night was the season's first frost. The campus lights shine through the pines around me, and the crackle of a frigid wood sounds from that cold darkness. I rub my hands together, breathe on them again, and place them in my jeans' pockets. Eventually, from the other side of the woods where the incoming road lies, headlights shine, and when my roommate pulls to the curb, I get in. Neither of us speaks as we drive down Market Street through downtown Wilmington and toward the Cape Fear River. The sky lightens, and by the time we unlock the boathouse and lay out the paddles for the rowers, the morning is a pale gray.

When the rowers arrive, we lug the boat to the riverside. The rowers grab underneath the shell's hull, and hoist it and carry it to the water where—there being no dock—it is rolled over and gently placed in the river while I give commands and follow along nearby. My bare toes sink into cold muck, squishing the sand, slime, and slick grit of the polluted river bottom, and the river soon numbs my feet beyond sensation. They feel thick as they knead the doughy river floor. I lower myself into the coxswain's position, knock my feet gently on the boat's tender side to shake mud from them and revitalize some feeling. Then we push out into the river that fogs with cold.

We row a four-man. Old, wooden, and not like the newer and lighter fiberglass models, it is heavy, but still we stroke through the smooth-top river. I call out the commands hastily taught to me, and the rowers laugh when I get a few wrong. But we row, and from the river's center I marvel at Wilmington's downtown streets and her historic waterfront.

As the temperature rises from frigid to just cold, plumes of vapor hover just above the river's surface while, nearby, the tread of cars crossing Memorial Bridge breaks the quiet. On the opposite shore an egret dives for food, dipping its beak close to where the battleship is permanently docked. Then there is the barge: moving heavy in the water, heading downriver on a course set to collide with our fragile skiff.

"We've got to get out of its wake," one of the rowers yells, panic visible on his back-turned face.

I shout out power strokes that require the men to use all their might, and, trying to outpower the other ship's mechanical motor, we stroke feverishly to the other shore. As the barge passes, the men use their oars to balance atop the large waves that curl from its bow and churn whitely from its stern. We rock dangerously, but keep our bodies centered, our minds focused, and soon the river calms again and the skiff no longer bobs. We are safe.

We row to a spot upchannel, an artery of the Cape Fear that is even calmer than the river herself. Here the men practice shifting in their seats, rolling to the catch, and flipping their oars for a smooth and strong pull in the water. We are silent: I hear the splash of water, the grunt of the rowers, the click of wooden oars slapping against wooden boat, and then the quiet flow of the river as we slip through it.

November 1991. It is after Thanksgiving. I've just returned from the family holiday and have been busy with papers and prepping for final exams. Sean—a freshman who rooms down the hall—sits across from me underneath Krispy Kreme's "Hot Now" sign as we both take a needed study break. His dark brown hair curls from the humidity and his amber eyes widen and dart around in a twitch. We eat doughnuts, sip coffee. Often this semester, we have come here: to sit, to eat, to talk. And though we have said much, I have not said enough. At least not until now.

"I've got something to tell you." And I begin: tell of my hemophilia, my HIV.

Sean stops eating his doughnut and brings both hands to his coffee cup's lid, where they fidget abstractly. Save for the sound of our breathing, it is quiet. I hear the rasp-heavy voice of a smoker ordering at the counter, the mellifluous trickle of a cup of coffee being poured, the click of a metal car door outside, the strain of the glass door being opened, the quiet laughter of a couple entering. I sip my coffee.

"That's heavy," Sean says. "Really heavy."

His finger traces the napkin's Krispy Kreme symbol as a child just learning to write. He stares into his coffee, looks outside the window, runs his hand through his hair, and breathes out heavy. "For what it's worth, I'm glad you told me . . . I'm not sure that I can help any, but if my knowing helps then I'm glad." He pauses, sips his coffee, sets it back on the tabletop. "But I've got a million questions, and I don't even know where to start. But one in particular is just nagging at me, and if it's too personal you can just tell me to go to hell." He stammers. "Ana? Does she know?"

"Yes. Of course."

"Wow. Okay. That's what I thought." His eyes roll around in thought. "You two are . . ." He hesitates, tilts his head. "You know . . . ?"

"Yes."

"And it's safe, right?"

"It's safe."

"Wow. I mean damn. I don't know what to say. What should I say? Is there anything to say? Hell, I don't even know how to act. This is really fucked up, you know. It's all fucked up." He looks to me. His eyes grow large with excitement and are bright and earnest in the fluorescent light. "You got fucked," he vociferates loudly. "You know that? I think I'd be in someone's face or something. I'd have to react. This is way too fucked up to not do something. I mean damn." Another coffee sip. "I always knew I'd learn about the world in college, but I didn't think it'd be like this. This is just plain fucked up. Damn." He sips again. "Sorry, man. This is just fucked up and I don't know what else to say but that." Slurp. "Fucked up."

The following afternoon when I return from my classes, I find Sean watching TV and smoking Camels. A big blue haze puffs around him, and as he turns to me, I can tell that he has not rested well. The dark skin beneath his eyes sags, and his disheveled hair appears as if his hands have been running through it all night, all day. Clothed in beer-mug boxers and a Charlotte Hornets T-shirt, he leans back into a chair marked by cigarette burns and beer stains. He nods hello as he shakes a cigarette out of the pack and tosses this onto the table where a pyramid of empty beer cans remains on display.

"I couldn't sleep last night," he says, lighting his cigarette. "I thought about you."

I drop my backpack and sit across from him. "I guess that you weren't expecting that kind of news about me last night."

"*That . . . That* was not what I expected." He pauses. "At all."

"I know."

He presses his cigarette butt into the ashtray and then flips another from his pack, taps it on the coffee table in front of him. "I don't know what I'm supposed to say about it." He brings the cigarette to his lips, lights it, and, when he exhales, I watch as smoke plumes from his mouth, clouding the distance between us. The scent of tobacco wafts toward me. "I've been smoking a shitload of these," Sean says, gesturing to his cigarette. "I don't know what else to do, so I just smoke and smoke a fuckload while crazy shit runs through my mind. A of all, I think about you and your having to deal with this shit and how fucked up that is, and then B of all I think about me, and, well, I'll be honest . . . I get a little scared."

"It's safe. I'm safe. And you're not in any danger."

"Well, I know that. At least on a logical level, but, man . . ." He exhales. "Still, it's making me fucking crazy. I mean, what if you were to cut yourself and bleed all over the place or something like that. That's some really crazy shit to think about. I really don't know what I'd do. I don't think that *would* happen, but just the thought that it could scares the piss out of me. . . . That's what this crazy head of mine has been doing to me all night. It creates these horrific situations and plays them out in my head, and it freaks the shit out of me." He puffs. Smoke fills the room. "I'm all fucked up. And I should be supporting you. I should be a better friend to you, and I feel like

I'm supposed to do something. Like I should drop out of school with you and tour the world or some fucked up shit like that. Oh God, I feel like one of those fucking movies." He leans his body forward and rests his head in his palms in a position of deep worry and concern.

"I hope you don't hate me for telling you. That's not what I meant."

Sean rights himself, pulls smoke into his lungs. "No. Certainly not. I've just gotta learn to deal. That's all. I've gotta deal."

He drags deeply on his cigarette. A wisp of smoke trails from his mouth. He coughs. "This smoking shit is really killing me, and I know I've gotta quit, but I can't today. It's keeping me sane."

December 1991. Inside my English professor's office, I sit as our conference begins. Her hair is wild and uncombed, and she tucks a mat of it behind her ears to reveal eyes tired from reading my class's essays. Papers are strewn across her desk, and rows upon rows of books line her walls and casket us in her office. She rustles her pile, retrieves a paper from it, and tosses it to me. I flip hastily through it, eventually arriving at the last page which has an A marked upon it.

"What's your major?"

"Marine biology," I answer with a certain lack of confidence. This was a thing I declared when I felt pressured into making myself a major of something. I reasoned that I loved fish, and so I would follow myself through a career with fish. Yet it isn't as I envisioned it. I'm not achieving high marks in my field, am not learning anything about fish, nor am I particularly enjoying it. I haven't even seen a fish since stepping on campus. I've studied mitochondria, DNA, RNA, the Golgi apparatus, and the convoluted insides of frogs, but no fish.

"Marine biology," the professor repeats. "Really. I'd have never guessed that." She aims her finger at my essay and I look down to again notice my A. "It's a good essay," she says. "A fine piece." And then she points her finger toward me. "You've got more a mind for English, I'm afraid. You should think about that. You should think about doing that."

"I'm flattered."

"Well, I meant to make you think about it, not flatter you."

"Okay. Then I'll think about it."

"Okay great. Think about it."

THROWING HOPE AWAY

FEBRUARY 1992. ANOTHER COLD WINTER MORNING. AT 6:00 A.M. rowing practice began, and now, at 8:30, I eat breakfast in the school cafeteria, enjoying a Belgian waffle with syrup. And later when I pedal to my nine o'clock literature class, my nausea comes on suddenly, and, having little time to react, I lean my head over the bike frame and throw up in the landscaped median. It is over quickly and is, thankfully, only witnessed by one student. I smile to him, wave that I'm okay, and continue to class. But before going, I splash water on my face in the bathroom and momentarily consider returning to my room for rest. Yet we have a test, I argue, and I feel okay. I should attend. I hold a wet paper towel to my forehead, inhale and exhale, assuring myself that I am well.

In class, I answer the short responses, concentrate on the essay question, and then my foot contracts in a spasm. I run my shoe along the floor, trying to press my foot flat within it and work my knot away. My foot twists. I breathe deeply, slowly, and concertedly to ease my pain, but it continues. I slip my shoe off, massage my foot through my sock, and feel the pain gradually subside. I flex my toes, stretch them out, and then return to my test. In the last months, the frequency of these spasms has steadily increased. And so has the nausea. I sense that something is wrong.

In the evening, I join Sean in the cafeteria. Having read some articles, called a few hotlines, and being assured that I am in more danger from HIV than him—he apologizes for his extreme reaction and states that he is no longer afraid of me. I say that I understand, that it isn't his fault, that the media has encouraged his response. We slap hands, high five, and then I load my plate with food, but upon sitting am immediately seized with spinning and nausea. I close my eyes and try to control myself.

"Are you okay?" Sean asks.

"Yeah. I'll be fine. I'm just not that hungry tonight."

I excuse myself and leave, bracing an arm against my stomach, another to my forehead. Outside, the wind throws the evergreen limbs around, and the sunlight that passes through them is as a strobe upon the sidewalk. My nausea increases. I fall into a nearby bench and feel the cold air chill the sweat beaded along my forehead. I shut my mouth to hold in my sickness. I breathe through my nose, listen at its sound rushing in and out of my nostrils, a noise like the wind swirling around me. Footsteps pass by. A girl asks another: *You think he's okay?* And then the wind gusts their voices away as flickers of sunlight dance across my eyelids and as the trees rustle overhead, producing a great whirling sky. When I force myself to stand, the wind catches my back and propels me forward.

In my room, I draw my trash can near and lie back and close my eyes. The room spins, my stomach quivers, and my body lightens as sick air against a mattress. I force my head into the trash can and heave until my deep gagging only yanks up sound and green spittle. My thin stomach muscles tighten; my throat roughens. I rest back and again close my eyes, and with my pillowcase, I catch the warm tears spilling from them. This cannot go on. This must stop.

In the night, another spasm wakes me. My left foot cramps like the parabolic arch of a scared cat's back—an arabesque of pain. To soothe it, I get out of bed and walk it off, hobbling round my room, stepping gingerly and occasionally flexing my toes to stretch my muscle. Outside, crickets sing their last song before the sun will soon rise, and the campus lights blaze in the dark courtyard—feeble orbs in a cloud of night. Eventually, my foot unlocks itself, and the pain fades. I lie down again.

Today it happens at lunch. My skin pales, my body warms, and my throat closes itself while my stomach churns. I push my food away and rush to my suite, where I give my insides to the toilet. Done, I lie down and sleep through another afternoon class, and later, I eat a slice of bread and wait to see that it stays down. Then, on what strength I have, I study. I'm behind in several classes now.

It is early morning, and I feel sick for the seventh time this week. My forehead sweats and my stomach roils. I go to the bathroom, hover over the open toilet, and wait for the spell to pass. I gag lightly, quietly, but nothing comes up. I run cold water over a cloth and press this to my face. It is cool and raises chill bumps along my arms as I sit on the bathroom floor and wait, and when the nausea ends, I return to my bed for a few more minutes of sleep, but soon I wake, dress for class, and swallow my AZT before leaving.

March. It has gone on for far too long. I cannot eat without food later spilling out of me, and I cannot walk without a muscle contraction striking me down. Now at four in the morning, I am bent prostrate in the suite bathroom, throwing my stomach into the toilet again. While the rest of the hall sleeps and while the first cool dew clings to the trees and grass outside, I am sick underneath the fluorescent light and its electric hum. I have no doubts that AZT causes this; research confirms it and my intuition tells me it is so. I wet my face with a cool washcloth. I wash my hands. I rinse my mouth with Listerine. And I return to bed, tiptoeing past my sleeping roommate.

When I wake again in another few hours, I shower, dress, and I then cup a cold glass of orange juice in one hand and palm the obligatory white and blue pill in the other. I hold it to the light, scrutinize the tiny particles encased in its shell, and wonder at it all. Twice a day, every day since I found out about my HIV, I have swallowed this pill unquestioningly. Today I pause. Although I have trusted AZT with my life, I think I can trust it no more. This is no way to live.

I walk into my room, the pill in hand, and I fetch the rest of the bottle, still hidden in my dresser drawer. I shake it and hear the rattle of the tiny, life-saving medicine within. Then, from where I'm standing at my bedside,

I make a long free-throw shot to the trash can. The bottle whacks against the concrete wall and banks in, making a tiny thump as it settles atop crumpled paper.

I don't call to consult Dr. Trum, for I can guess his advice. He has his numbers to believe in. He has his charts and his faith in medicine. I don't ask my mother or my father what they think, for, just as AZT is my only hope, so it is theirs, and I can't ask them to give up a thing like that. So for now, I take this upon myself. I am sick of being sick.

I remove the trash bag from the can and ponder the AZT bottle one last time before hauling it to the dumpster. Outside, a cool breeze blows the stink of trash toward me, and I again feel nauseous as I hurl the bag over the container's top. The bag flies up and hovers momentarily before descending and crashing against the metal inside. When I hear the heavy thud of it settling, the crackling of glass, the woofing exhale of foul air—I cross my fingers and wish for strength and health immeasurable. I need a miracle now. A Merlin to save me.

April. Friday night, Ana and I attend a keg party in a house off Walker Street in Greensboro, and our spirits are lifted with drink. We laugh heavily as we hold hands and totter our way back to Ana's dorm where we have sex like two drunk lovers having sex. We slur I love you until intoxication sends us dreams. We sleep until, several hours later, daylight brightens her room and wakes us. Ana rises to close her blinds and returns with glasses of cold water. I drink. She drinks. Then we adjust her covers and sleep more.

We wake in the late afternoon, order burgers from a local grill, and watch a matinee at the nearby cinema, and when we return to her dorm, we are both still tired from the night before. Ana rests her arms across my chest as her room darkens with night. She is almost asleep.

"I've quit it, Ana," I say to her sleeping face. She opens her eyes, lifts her head from her pillow.

"Quit what?"

"The AZT."

She stills her hand over my heart.

"I'm so scared," she says.

"I am, too."

"What will you do? Isn't there anything else? Isn't there any way to take it? Is it really making you that sick?"

"It's done. There is nothing else to do but wait."

She lays her face against my cheek. "Oh, I hate this," she says. "I hate this."

I hear the patter of footsteps along the corridor outside, the giggle of girls, and then this fades. Ana turns back to me.

"It's your decision," she says softly. "I guess I have to trust you."

She squeezes against me, trails her finger against my backbone. We fumble our hands together and press hope against our palms. We kiss in the dark.

When I return to Wilmington on Sunday, a lifting storm lets the sun poke through the clouds, warming the earth, and, not ready to return to school and its many demands, I head to the beach. I drive past the azaleas blooming along Airlie Road and crest the bridge over the Atlantic water-way to descend into a landscape of estuaries, sea grass, and vacation homes constructed where land allows. Parking near the Trolley Stop, I buy two of their mustard and cheese Surfer dogs and eat these outside where gulls wing around me in a white flutter.

Later I walk along the beach. The gulls escort me, cawing to and fro, and, rooted to nothing, they are borne aloft by the sea's constant breeze. I follow the sands north to Mercer's Pier and spend money on a rusty pin-ball machine. I feed the game quarters, trying to keep the ball alive, but I lose quickly. The fishermen and their long poles come and go, and a few drag vines of sea bass with them. A ball slips past my flipper, the lights stop flashing, the pinball's siren quiets, and another game ends. I count my change and consider breaking a few more dollars, but instead I pocket those not yet spent.

Outside, clouds balance upon the marine-blue sea, and beside the pier, I gaze out to an ocean bleeding into a vermillion sky. A woman and her dog jog past: he breathing hard, tongue slapping out his open mouth; intent upon moving forward, they are immune to the view.

The sea washes my feet as the waves spread foam across a slick of sand. The wooden pilings labor to hold up a blood-red sky. Night descends.

June. In the blood-drawing lab, the phlebotomist plumps my arm with her tourniquet, and soon my stout veins run in vague blue streams from my elbow to my finger joints.

"Wow," the phlebotomist remarks. "You've got great veins. It's not often I see a set like that. Like mountain chains."

"I guess if you're going to be a hemophiliac, you should come with good veins."

She laughs lightly as she lines up small purple-, red-, blue-, and orange-topped tubes. After the blood collection, the tubes are spun and the blood tabulated, and today I wonder what the numbers will say. I wonder how my decision to stop AZT will affect that count.

The phlebotomist swipes my arm with the alcohol swab, feels her finger along a vein in my forearm.

"Please don't bruise it," I say, as she slips her silver-tip needle into me. "I need all the good veins I can get." Often, the oversized needles the doctors use leave my veins blown and complicate my home treatment. Blood flows into the clear tubing and into the test vials. I watch it; the nurse watches it; the tubes fill.

When I am done, I meet Mom in the lobby. She rode up with me from New London, where I'm staying over the summer break. She wanted to be a mother today, she had said the night before, and she wanted to visit the doctor with me, like she used to do, she added. I did not object.

"All done?" she asks with her general cheerfulness.

"Yep."

Through the long white corridor as we return to the hemophilia clinic, I tell Mom about stopping AZT. She shakes her head in concern and disappointment.

"I don't understand. You just quit it?"

"Yes."

"And Dr. Trum thought it was best?"

"I'm telling him today."

"Oh, Son," she says. "Oh, Son, no."

We keep walking.

While we wait in the clinic, we toss magazine pages by and pass the time in silence. Here, in *People*, everyone looks so happy. In my lap lies a pile of endless smiles.

"Shelby Smoak," a nurse calls.

"That's me," I answer while rising to be ushered to my examination room.

And later when Dr. Trum enters, my mom blurts out that I've stopped taking AZT.

"He just told me this morning," she says as I swing my legs over the table's side. "Even his father doesn't yet know. I can't believe he's done this without telling us." She looks at me. "I can't believe you've done this and put yourself at such danger while leaving us all in the dark, especially Dr. Trum. He's the specialist here."

Dr. Trum joins in: "You should really thoroughly consider what you've done. Of course, as your doctor, I'll support your decision and treat you as best as I can, but without taking AZT our options are limited. I just want you to understand that this isn't like stopping Tylenol."

"If it's the nausea," Mom says, "Dr. Trum says he can give you something for it."

"Yes. We can treat the side effects."

"No," I say, with a confused conviction that I stand by. "There's the cramps, my inability to eat, the headaches, the throwing up . . . My decision is made. I can't go back on it. I felt far too lousy those last months, and I can't imagine it will get any better."

"But, Son," Mom says. "This is . . . This is . . ." She tries to maintain composure, but trembles and grabs a tissue from her purse and dabs her eyes to catch the tears while Dr. Trum rustles his papers.

"Please, please, stay in touch with me and this clinic," he says, addressing me. He frowns. "We need to work together on this. We're here to help you. Always remember that."

Mom blows her nose.

When Dr. Trum finishes his examination and before we are sent on our way, he once again expresses his grave concern about my decision. The room quiets, as there is nothing more to say.

Outside, the wind blows an April downpour upon us as Mom and I hurry to the parking deck. We are soaked, and as I shake the rain loose from my hair, Mom begins again:

"What if you get sick now? What if you get a cold . . . or worse? What then?"

"I just think I'm better off without AZT. That's no way to live."

"But medicine has always saved you. Just look at your factor and what it's done." We reach the car and dip inside and fasten our belts and begin to drive off.

"You know I love you, Son, and I just want you to be well. That's all I ever want. I'm not going to cry anymore to you about this, but I really don't agree with it. I wish you'd reconsider."

"Mom, I just can't live like that. That's not living."

"But I'm worried."

"And I'm worried, too."

We exit the parking deck into a clap of thunder and a dark sky falling with blue rain. I steer past the flooded hog lots and soaked meadows with the wipers squeaking along the windshield.

I am lost in the thought of my life hanging in the balance; only hope swaddles me, for there is nothing other than AZT to save me.

THE SPLIT

September 1992. Junior year. Another heat wave has left the coast, dragging its humidity across the southern sands; now the temperature peaks in the high eighties instead of the nineties. I swim in the Atlantic where the water is cool enough to enjoy and not yet cold enough to prohibit entering it. I let the waves buoy me and allow the tide to tell me where to go.

Last night Ana had called and said that she had found a ride to Wilmington for the weekend, and I suddenly felt a greater distance between us than our geography, for I told her to stay in Greensboro. I was busy; friends were coming to visit. We had had our summer together, and now I wanted more time for myself. I had explained this to her as we lay together on her parents' couch at the end of summer, but I could tell that my feelings were not hers. She sobbed. She bleated that she missed me. And I tried to explain that I only wished to spend more time alone; that it had nothing to do with her, or our relationship; that I felt as if my time was a grain of sand sifting through a giant sieve; that I needed to be with me. But she did not understand then. And that is how we left it. Until last night. And now she's upset.

A roll of water buoys me. My feet lift from the sea floor. I drift along with the current: as aimless and unguided as the ocean sand that is pushed to shore and then pulled out again with the ebbing tide.

William, visiting for the weekend, rises from his beach towel, strokes out to meet me, and stretches his body flat against the undulating water. He kicks into a coming wave. We swim. A brunette girl sunning herself on a float paddles nearby, and William asks me if I know her from school.

"No," I say.

"Well, I wish you did."

"Me, too. She's pretty."

"But you'll know some girls at this keg party tonight, right?"

"Probably. At least a few from my classes."

"And Ana? What about her? She coming?"

"No. Not tonight."

"Really?" William paddles on his back. "I'm surprised. I bet you miss her right now. I bet you think about her all the time."

"I don't."

"Ah . . . come on. You're a romantic. You can admit it. You believe all that stuff you read." William swims in a circle.

"Most of what I read isn't all that happy and romantic. It's sad and full of desolation. Fitzgerald, for example. Besides, I think Ana and I are breaking up."

William pauses his backstroke, treads water. "Breaking up?"

"Well, yeah. I told her I needed time for myself . . . Space."

"Ahhh. That's one thing you should never tell a girl if you wanna get her pants off."

"Ha-ha. I just think I need to focus more on myself, my studies. It was getting too serious, and I wasn't ready for that. Not yet. Mostly it just boils down to the fact that my feelings are not the same as hers. Not anymore."

"Does she know?"

"Well . . . I told her we're taking a little break, but we didn't 'officially' break up, I guess."

"Oh . . . Falling out of love, are you?"

"Maybe. Hard to say. Just taking time to figure it all out."

"Well, man. I'm sorry it ain't all roses, but I haven't heard of a relationship yet that is. Anyway, forget about it. Maybe your two's time has passed. Try and let yourself feel free and lose some of that lead baggage you're always dragging around with you. The sooner you make a decision about it, however, the better off both of you will be."

"I know, I know. It's just tough. It's hard to know what to do."

"Life's tough, man. You just gotta decide and move forward."

"I hear you."

William rides a wave to shore, and, climbing out of the sea, he props up again on his towel next to Sean and opens another beer from our cooler. I float on my back, feel the warm sun on my stomach, and listen to the swish of water in my ears. The flat sea shimmers, a giant sheen of metal.

When I lie on my towel, my body drips ocean. Sean opens the cooler, passes me a beer. "Come on, man. You gotta have more than one," he says.

And as I accept the beer and press the cold can to my forehead and roll it along my face, I understand that we are true pals again.

"It's for drinking, motherfucker."

"I know. It feels good, though."

I open it, swallow, and watch the day: the sun paused overhead; the waves spreading in an endless foam of white; the gulls wheeling round in an empty sky; and a couple tossing a Frisbee back and forth, their bodies statues with an occasional toss of the arm.

A girl in a two-piece passes nearby. We sip our beer and watch.

"I'd do her," William says before taking a long draft from his can.

"Maybe. But she's got a skinny ass. Nice tits, though."

Their eyes follow her as she walks down the beach, where she is replaced by a group of three girls.

"Oh, yeah. The one in the middle. I'd do her. No question."

"In your dreams," Sean says. "I'd do her first. Then her red-haired friend. Then both of them at the same time."

"As if . . ."

I sip my beer, watch another suntanned blonde pass. "I'd do her," I say, pointing with my can.

Sean and William look. "Oh yeah. There you go. Major hottie," Sean says.

Autumn.

"Remember me?" Ana sobs over the phone line. I imagine her at the other end: sitting cross-legged atop her bed, twirling the cord around her unsure hand. Her blonde hair is pulled back in a ponytail and a box of Kleenex rests in her lap.

She blows her nose, clears her sorrow.

"Of course I remember you. Don't be silly."

"Well, I haven't seen you all semester, so I wasn't sure. Am I still your girlfriend?"

"I don't know, Ana. I'm not anybody else's boyfriend if that's something."

"That's nothing. It just feels like you don't know." She pauses, blows her nose again. "So, are you coming to see me over fall break?"

"Yes, Ana. Tomorrow. I'll be there."

"Okay." A sniffle. "I miss you."

"I miss you too."

And when Ana hangs up, I drive to the ocean.

The sea is tumultuous; the sky dark with rain. It bellows and foams and sprays and is stirred to life by an offshore storm. Soon, a hurricane is expected: Category 3 with landfall in a few days. Residents await to hear about evacuations. And now everything seems so delicate, so fragile. I witness how the sea—so calm and pacific days ago—is now pitching and yawing with uncertainty; how a quiver of rain is only the veil before the whirling drape of a hurricane.

The pier lights disappear into a simpering sky. A lone surfer struggles against a crashing sea before he is swallowed and then spit out closer to shore. Before long, the rain begins and drives me to shelter in my truck, where I sit and watch the sky spark and alight with zags of lightning. All is in an uproar.

The following day, through the wind and the rain, I drive to see Ana. I've dreaded this moment: my heart tightens, my hands sweat; my anxiety dizzies me. I try to focus on the speech I will give. For days, I've rolled it over in my mind: how once, I loved her dearly. I loved her for doling out her love to me, for I imagine her love for me as a sacrifice, she throwing her body upon mine as upon a burning pyre. And I called this the ultimate love. But now I cannot breathe for it. The air between us is polluted by my own thoughts. How it has come to this, I cannot say exactly, but now my heart is empty and cannot be filled by her. I am ending our relationship.

It happens in her dimly lit dorm in the quiet of the weekend night. We are on her bed, where we often spooned our bodies tight together and made promises of hope and love. But now it is different.

"I don't understand," Ana weeps.

"I don't understand, either. It has just happened."

"What has happened? You don't love me anymore?"

"I don't know. Something has changed in me. It's me. I know it's me. I'm so sorry."

"But I trusted you. I put all I had in you." Ana sobs and sniffles as tears pour from her eyes and then she rushes from the room, leaving me to wonder how to react. I twist my hands together. Play with my thumbs. If I could yank out the guilt crushing my heart, I would.

When Ana reappears with a box of tissues, she sits at the opposite end of her bed, slumps into its corner, and curls her feet beneath her while blowing her nose, wiping her eyes.

"And you waited until you came here to tell me." She clears her nose again. "Why? Answer me that," she flares out. "Why?"

"I don't know. I didn't want to do it over the phone."

"Oh, you're a real gentleman . . . Is that all you can say?" Ana rights herself. "Is there someone else?" she asks. "Have you met someone else?"

"No. There's no one else."

"Are you sure?"

"Yes. This has everything to do with me . . . There's no one else."

Ana places her hair behind her ear and wipes her eyes, and I feel the event I've set in motion. The end of this, of something. My heart sinks into a hollow pit beneath my lungs, and I feel the sudden, gripping fear of loneliness.

"Maybe I don't know what I'm doing," I offer in a moment of retraction. "I've just had so many pressures on me at school, and it's been hard to keep seeing you."

"I don't think I ask for much."

"I know." I am forgetting about all those times I thought differently.

"I know you don't ask for much, but it's the idea of it. Perhaps I still need space. I want to be able to concentrate only on the things that are at school."

Ana grips the tissue between her hands. She moves closer and leans herself against me, and I instinctively put my arms around her. "We can take more space if that's what you need," she bargains. "This is just too much to take in at one time, and we shouldn't rush into things too quickly. Besides, I have my own studies and now that I'm working within my major, things are really busy for me, too."

"I don't know. I'm not so sure." I'm growing scared and fear blots out my clarity. Who else can love me as Ana has? Who can accept my HIV? Who?

"We can take some space, become more like friends. If this is what you need, I can do it," she pleads.

We kiss. She inhales, then sighs out heavily, and rests herself into my open arms. I can feel darkness around me. Everything is unsure, nothing is decided.

"Well," Ana says, tracing her finger along my hand, "what kind of friends do you think we should be?"

"I don't know." I feel the past revive itself. I remember love, happiness, sex.

"There's all kinds of friendships, you know."

Ana places her hands underneath my shirt and kisses me along my neck. And soon, we are slipping out of our clothes as if nothing has changed. We cleave to one another, are caught up in the natural grip of desire. And I let it happen, for it is easier this way.

Afterwards, neither of us has the courage to speak. There are no words to frame here, but only an awkward feeling. I cower beneath her sheets. I stare at her ceiling. I make a feeble attempt at placing my arms around her.

"You don't have to hold me," she says.

"I want to."

And she lets me. But now we have dressed up our relationship as a new friendship, a dreadful thing to do.

"Were you planning on staying the night?" Ana asks as I settle my heavy heart beside her.

"I wasn't sure. I hadn't thought things through."

"But you are now?"

"Yes. I'm staying tonight."

Ana flips on the television. "I'll order pizza," she says.

And the familiar comforts us, persuades our hearts away from notions of ruin and decay.

When the weekend ends, Ana walks me to the parking lot. I cast my eyes to the ground, and we do not link hands as we drift through the courtyard of fallen leaves. They lie in piles of dying color: orange sassafras, scarlet maple, yellow poplar, and maroon sweetgum. Blown by the wind, they leave the trees exposed to the coming cold. We proceed down the campus walk, coming eventually to the gravel lot and my small truck. I unlock my cab door, settle my bag within, and turn to Ana.

"So is this it?" she asks. "Is this where you say your good-bye? Or will I see you again?"

I absently draw my foot through gravel.

"I don't know, Ana. I'm not so sure this friendship thing is going to work out."

"No," she cries out. "Don't do this. Not like this." I try to reach for her, but she deflects me with her hand. "Stay away. Just stay away if that's how you want it." She wipes her eyes. "What was this, some kind of conjugal visit? Is that what this weekend was about? Is that what I was good for?"

"Ana, please. This isn't how I wanted it."

"No. No. You're an asshole! Fuck you!" A flock of sparrows riffles from the elm trees and instinctively, I turn and watch—a flap of black in a clouded autumn sky. "Just fuck you!" she yells again.

"But Ana, please!"

She runs off, arms flailing at her side. "Fuck you, you asshole!"

I fold my hands over my eyes and tears spill out. And this is how it ends: in hate.

SUMMER 21

MAY 1993. MOM, DAD, AND I ARRIVE AT MY SUMMER RESIDENCE IN downtown Wilmington. It is an enormous house set on a small lot with the neighboring homes bearing in upon it from the sides. We walk in and up the stairs guarded on the stout banister by carved owls, and on the top landing, we follow the slender hallway to where it spills onto a petite balcony; the backyard unfolds in summer green and is bound on three sides by a uniform wooden fence painted in colonial white, a landscape that momentarily transports me to another time.

We retrace our steps down the hall to a shut door that I slip open, revealing a dwarfish room.

"This is it," Mom says. "This can't be much more than a glorified broom closet with a window."

"But you can't beat a hundred dollars a month."

"If it's the money, Son, we can help you out. What about your roommates? How much are they paying?"

"I don't know, Mom. Maybe two, three hundred. It doesn't matter, though. This is what I can afford." I look around, breathe in. "And besides, I like it all right."

"How is he going to stand living here without air conditioning?" Mom asks, addressing Dad. "How?"

Dad looks around, doesn't answer.

"I'll be fine, Mom. It's only for a few months anyway."

"You're just going to have to accept that our son's growing up," Dad says to Mom.

"Well, I don't like it," she says to Dad. "You need to take care of yourself," she then says to me. "Don't forget that. Your health always comes first."

"I won't forget it. I'll be fine."

She miffs her face, raises her hands in a gesture of exasperation. "Okay. Fine. Let's move you in."

For the duration of the afternoon, we unload my belongings, and when Mom leaves to get the last of my things from the car, Dad knocks a cigarette from his pack and lights it. He leans over to catch his breath and then rights himself again. "Your mom's just upset because I'm not going to be home this summer, either."

"You're not? Why not? What's going on?"

"The plant in town's not doing good. I'm pretty sure it's going under, so I'm getting out while I still have a chance."

"I don't understand. What are you going to do?"

"Well, Son, I called a friend, and I'm going to be consulting for a few factories. I'll move from place to place and show them how to set up the fabric cutters so they can save money."

"But where?"

"Actually, here. Wilmington. It's my first job."

"Wilmington? You're going to be here this summer?"

"Yes. Your mom and I didn't want to tell you because, well . . . we just found out, and I knew we were coming here and could just tell you then."

"Wow. I'm shocked." I spread my clothes out along my mattress. "So when do you start?"

"Two weeks."

"And the bills? You and Mom can still pay them?"

"That's got your mom a bit on edge," Dad says, breathing out another puff of smoke. "But I think we're going to be fine."

Mom returns with the final box of my clothes, bracing her hands underneath it.

"Where do you want this?" she asks, a bit winded from her ascent. "It doesn't look like it'll fit in that closet of yours, but you need to be careful with it. The bottom's about to fall out."

"Out there in the hallway is fine," I say. She lowers the box to the floor and slides it against the wall.

"Did you tell him?" Mom asks Dad, who quickly answers that he did. "I'm not too happy about it," she says to me, "but I'm just glad that maybe you two will get to see one another. Dad's suppose to check to make sure you're eating right and not starving in this cave."

"Think of it like Plato's cave. From within, I'll contemplate the world."

"Ha-ha. The true scholar, eh?"

Together, we unpack a few more boxes until my room is soon full and we agree that we can fit no more. There's space for a mattress, clothes, a few books, CDs, and a small TV-tray where I place my jambox. The bed is just comfortable enough and the room sufficiently good. I remove the rest of my items to a storage space underneath the stairwell, one that Dad claims outsizes my own room. Then we sit on the front porch and sip glasses of cool water as a warm breeze blows through the downtown avenue. We let out our fatigue and take in the homes and their historic architecture.

After a while, Dad shuffles his feet and reaches over to pat Mom on her hand.

"Well," he says, "I reckon we should get going, let our son get settled in and let us start the drive home."

And so they gather up and Dad cools the car while we say good-bye underneath the river birches and summer magnolias.

"It's gonna be hard not even having you home this summer," Mom says. "You all grow up so fast." She hugs me and slips me some money. "This is to help with that first month. I wish I could give you more, but as it is, things with your dad's job are already uncertain."

"Are you sure you can afford this?"

"Yes. It's okay. You take that. Pay your rent and use the little that's left to buy yourself some food. You're looking awfully thin and you won't be home for me to fatten you up."

We hug again as the heat presses on us, the sun blazing in the sky.

"Good-bye. We'll miss you." She gets in the car next to Dad. "Be sure you come visit when you're not working."

"I will."

And they leave.

Exhausted from the move, I return to my room and flip on the box fan and fall into the mattress, which rests on the floor, and soon the lazy heat and the long day have their effects, and I fall asleep.

In the blood lab at UNC Hospitals, I relinquish my arm to the phlebotomist. She tells me there's going to be a little stick, and then she punctures me, draws her tubes of blood, and sends me down the corridor to wait for Dr. Trum. He flexes my joints, listens to life in my chest, and consults numbers in my chart.

"And you're not going back on the AZT?" he inquires noncommittally.

"No."

"Your numbers *are* going down. I'll get your labs back from today and compare, but I think come winter we may start you on a pneumonia prophylaxis. Think you can handle that?"

"Sure. Okay."

"It'll lessen your chances of getting sick."

When I leave his office, I submit next to the orthopedist's examination—he still expresses concern about my hip's decline and admonishes me for failing to use a cane—and then done, I leave and park along Franklin Street, which never fails to interest me. The summer scholars cradle books while they await the trundling roar of the coming bus. Passersby pause before store windows and point to items they wish to own. An elderly florist sits in a small stretch of building shade, huddling round her garden of flowers— flashes of natural color in a concrete sea. And the jeweler toddles round the large black clock marking his store, roving his carefree head around and occasionally checking his own wristwatch for the time.

At noon, the street lunches. The hot dog vendor fishes long slips of red wieners with his tongs, and he places these in steamed buns and dresses them with ketchup, mustard, onions, slaw, and chili. Nearby, patrons line the inside glass front of a small bistro and prop at undersized tables, taking petite bites of sandwiches made with breads of rye, sourdough, and sun-dried tomato.

I enter the drugstore and lunch at the counter. On one side of me, a lady in a blue dress swirls a fry in a dab of ketchup. On the other side, a cop calls out to the cook and says that he made an arrest earlier, that it was a college basketball star, and that it would appear on the nightly news. The cook momentarily turns away from his grill of sizzling burgers, says, "No shit" to the cop, and then begins to flip the hamburgers one by one, soon setting them onto buns garnished with lettuce and tomato.

"I'll have one of those," I say to the counter waitress. "No cheese. Fries. And a Coke to drink." And when the food arrives, I eat, surrounded by smiling photographs of former patrons.

Across the street is a record store, and when I'm finished eating, I go there, thumb through the new releases, finger the few bills in my pocket, and leave without a purchase. I stroll a few blocks west to enter a bookshop. The stacks tower over me with books whose tattered covers promise me the world. I loosen one from the shelf and unfold it to a page of faded ink. And before its printing, I think, it was the blue ink run from a pen and set down upon a sleeve of antique-laid paper, for this is how I imagine all writers work: with fountain pens, ink bottles, and thick paper. From the store window, light peeks down the aisle and shines upon the dust motes floating midair between James and Joyce. I run my finger along the hubbed spine of one, feel the antique luxury of leather, but pass on, buying instead a worn Graham Greene paperback.

Outside in the sun again, I read the first paragraph. They are beautiful phrases, rhythmic and true. I linger at a table outside a coffee shop, drink caffeine, and imbibe the world in my hand. Nearby, a group of girls chatters, tossing their hair in fits of laughter. More girls invade the area. And they are all so beautiful with their blue and green and hazel eyes flaring in the sunlight. I stare at one in a pink top. She stares back. I smile. She smiles. My heart flutters.

For money, I work at Fort Fisher: site of a famous Civil War battle and a place that beachgoers often stumble into when their sunburns are too great or when a downpour closes the beach. I give tours, answer questions, sell merchandise. Erected on the Cape Fear River's mouth, this fort protected the South, guarded Wilmington, and shielded the Confederate troops inside its man-made sand mounds, which were built atop boxed wooden structures. Atop these mounds, soldiers placed lookouts and mounted cannons while they kept a fearful eye toward the river, the sea, and the Northern blockade. They constructed a ten-foot fence around them to guard against land invasion, and through the slats, they fired muskets at scavenging squirrels as practice targets for the coming battle. But all that is now gone. The fence is a reconstruction, and the sandy hills are overrun with a century of growth where Sandburg's grass is, indeed, doing its work.

Along the fort's beach, live oaks arch backwards as if reaching their hands for the river behind them. Bent by endless ocean winds and low to the ground, their branches offer an easy perch where I have lunch, enjoying a quiet view of the sea while the salt breeze keeps the summer's heat from scorching me. Down the slope of sand and onto the beach, the gentle lap of waves murmurs against a shore whose blood was born away more than a century before I was born.

June. In the early evening when the colors soften and the heat cools and the day's work has been done, I meet Dad at the Oceanic Pier. It is his first week of work in Wilmington, and, anxious to swim, he is there and already wet when I arrive.

"I can't believe you didn't wait on me," I say, approaching him.

"It was too hot." He stands to hug me. "I had to cool off."

I lay my towel next to his, remove my shirt and shoes.

"I'm going in," I say, striding down the ocean bank to the sea. Dad follows, and we wade out beyond the breakers, bobbing in salt water as the afternoon latens. We catch the occasional wave to shore, riding our inherited thin, flat chests as boards. And afterwards, we dry on our towels, the sun heating our backs as we stare toward the sea's horizon.

"How are you?" Dad asks, still gazing at the ocean and the fading day. He shakes a Marlboro from the pack, lights it. Smoke curls from his nicotine-yellowed hands, spews from his mouth and nose.

"Fine," I say. We don't talk about HIV.

"Job working out okay?"

"Yes. I'm paying the bills at least."

"Mom and I will help out some, but it's time you started learning to make your own way in the world. Next year's the year."

"Yeah. I know."

"Do you know what you're gonna do?"

"I'm figuring it out." I run my hands along my legs, knocking off sand. I haven't thought much about graduating from college, it still seeming far away, and long-term planning being anathema to HIV, so for now, I try to enjoy this summer. Life's easier this way.

"Well, don't let it sneak up on you. You're gonna need a good job. And you're gonna need insurance." Dad looks to me. "You can't live without insurance, Son."

I nod that I understand. And I do. I'm just not ready for those concerns. Most fathers must talk to their sons like this, but his hammering of insurance scares me.

Dad rubs a cigarette into the sand, taps his yellowed hands along thin damp legs while the shadows of our bodies stretch down the sloped embankment and almost to the water. The sun is low; the tide is high.

"You coming home anytime soon?" Dad asks, breaking the sound of the waves and my thoughts in them.

"Soon, yes. But not this weekend. There's a birthday party for me. Maybe the next."

"Your mom misses you. She's going to have a hard time with Anne leaving for college this year, too."

"I know, but my life is here. In Wilmington." I brush a sandy hand on my towel.

"I know, Son. It's just a lot of changes for your mom at once. Me working out of town. Anne starting school. And you, not coming home for the summer. Go see her. You can ride with me one weekend."

"I will. I promise I will."

"Your mom wants to see you. She misses you."

We sit a while longer on our towels, letting the constant wind dry us.

People stroll in front of us while the lights of the Oceanic begin to shine more brightly and the restaurant bustles with diners eager for seafood. When the sky becomes its late-day violet, we scoop our towels from the beach, shake them off, and begin walking toward our cars.

"How about the same time next week?" Dad asks.

"As long as there's no rain, that sounds great. It's a perfect time for a swim, tourists gone and it not too hot."

When we near Dad's car, he opens his door and pulls a card from his seat. "Here," he says. "Since we won't be seeing you this weekend, it's an early birthday present. It's just a bit of money," he says as I open the card and see the cash, "but we thought that you could get a good dinner somewhere."

"Thanks, Dad."

"Mom's got something else for you, but you know you'll have to come home for that. She's not gonna mail it or send it by me."

"That sounds like her," I laugh. "I'll be home soon. I promise."

"Happy birthday, Son," Dad says, giving me a farewell hug.

And as he drives away into the fading purple, nostalgia overcomes me. I have grown up and moved out of the house. And it all happened so quickly.

June 9. Sean and I drive to the store to get the keg for tonight's party, and in the parking lot, he shoves me a wad of green bills, commenting that everyone should buy a keg on their twenty-first birthday. Inside, the lady behind the counter asks for my ID, and I proudly produce it. She is old and wrinkled, her eyes a pruned topography of skin.

"Oh, happy birthday," she says, coughing out of a phlegmatic lung while taking the cash I give her.

"Thanks."

Another employee brings out the keg on a dolly, and I roll this outside and down the handicap ramp.

"Aren't you going to help?" I ask of Sean, who idles in my truck's cab. "This thing's heavy and I can't lift it myself." He flips open his passenger door.

"Sorry, dude. I can't touch it. I'm still twenty." He laughs, saunters over, and hoists the keg into my truck bed. "Pussy," he chides.

Later, my house parties. Gleaming candles are set around the place, flickering in the corners and dancing shadows upon the walls. In the great room, the stereo booms, growing louder as the night lengthens. Two lines form along the hallway: one for the restroom, the other for the keg iced down on the small balcony. But really, one line is an extension of the other. A cup is filled, is drunk, and is then pissed out to make room for another. At least this is how I begin to see the night as I revolve from keg to toilet and so on.

The party is a good-looking crowd. The fit captain of the crew team swings his arm around a cherub-faced teacher in training; a lithe basketball scholar proves his athleticism by performing several keg stands; and a steady couple brings their argument to the party, making loud overtures of their hate for one another. Several beers into the night, however, a partygoer discovers this same couple in my roommate's bedroom and snaps paparazzi photographs of their naked embarrassment. We laugh. They laugh, they blush.

I lay my eye upon Portia—a striking redhead with a wide and easy grin—and I absently trail her from room to room. For a time we dance together, but when she later hooks herself to a boy in a buttoned blue shirt, I give up the pursuit and find something else to occupy me. I chat with friends. I play songs on the stereo.

By 3:00 A.M., the keg is dry and the party disperses. Two bodies with open mouths drinking in the inebriated night air sprawl on the couch; another several have passed out on the floor; and my roommates' rooms are all occupied as well. I crawl through my second-story window and sit on the rooftop, pondering the few stars visible through the streetlights' fluorescent glow. A cool breeze rustles the nearby trees while farther away, the crickets harmonize in the night. A car shoots out of the dark, rambles along the avenue, and beams light on the night-silver trees. Soon Sean steps out of my window to join me.

"So, this is where you're off to. Hiding out on the roof."

"I'm not hiding. I just felt like being here." The smell of the river drifts in the wind and mingles with the fragrance of gladiolas. A light fog puffs about us. "Twenty-one," I tell Sean as he lowers himself beside me. "Twenty-one."

"I know." He nods his head, tips back his beer cup. "And you're doing great."

"I am."

We sit quietly. Below us a man bicycles past, pedaling in the night.

"I got a letter this week. A birthday card from Ana."

Sean sips his beer. "Really," he says. "How's she doing?"

"Well, it wasn't exactly from her. It was from an AIDS organization, PWA. It says that she's made a donation in my name, honoring my birthday." Sean, staring off past the elm tree that shades the front lawn, brings the beer to his lips again and takes a long draw. "Can you believe that? It was a lot of money, too." Sean nods. "I can't believe it. I guess that even after all the hurt I caused her, I can at least feel like she doesn't want me dead." And then it is out there, the brutal irony.

Sean and I can't control ourselves. We laugh loudly. I hold my side and lie flat onto the rooftop to catch air, and it is good.

"That's great," Sean says. "That's really something, you know."

"I know. I can't even say how it made me feel."

"So, did you tell anyone about it?"

"No. And I'm not going to. This is just something I'll keep to myself."

"Your secret's safe with me," he says as he stands. He sips again. "So I'm heading back in and will leave you to your thoughts. Besides, I've got this little hottie that I think may go home with me." He ducks back through the window. "Don't stay out here too long trying to solve all the world's problems tonight," he shouts back before a long silence returns and the crickets chirp in the background.

A few minutes later, Sean yells up to me from the front yard, says, "I'm headin'."

"Later," I call back. A young blonde is leashed to his arm and they both stumble to his car.

"She's cute," I call out.

"Hey. What'd ya expect?" he says throwing up his arms and letting out a laugh that echoes through the quiet street.

Sean falls into his car seat, cranks, swerves away, and howls out his window as he speeds down the avenue. I watch the taillights fade.

Later, the stereo quiet, the lights out, the party over—I slip back through my window and fall into my mattress, listening to the box fan hum a sleepy breeze.

At a club in downtown Wilmington, I meet Kaitlin. She dances, and as I watch her twirl to the music, I pine for the happiness that she exudes. A few songs later when she notices me smiling, she stops dancing, sidles to the bar next to me. I drink to increase my courage and to slow my nervous heart. I give her a hard stare.

"Can I buy you a drink?"

"No," she says. "I think I've had enough tonight." She curls threads of chestnut hair behind her ear and stares at the dancers still swaying on the floor.

"Okay. Fair enough." My palms sweat. My heart pounds. "What if I just sit here and drink for you while we talk."

"Sure, okay. But I'm getting ready to leave."

I take another sip. "Or I could just get your phone number and see if you're interested in going out sometime?"

She turns to look at me, her hazel eyes bright in the darklight. "Boy, you just cut to the chase don't you?"

I shrug my shoulders. "I think it's the alcohol talking. I'm usually the shy guy you'd never meet."

"Sure you are. That's okay. You don't have to lie." She opens her purse, pulls out a notepad, writes a number on it, tears a sheet off, folds it, and passes it to me. "Here. Here's your number." I read it aloud.

"Is this real? It doesn't sound like a real number. There's too many fives."

"Guess you'll just have to call it to find out," she says as she stands to leave. She gives me a playful wave and slips away.

I polish off my drink and play the scrap of paper between my fingers much as if I were twirling a flower.

Walking home, I pause before a house's bay window and listen to a piano echoing from within. The sound, soft and distant, haunts the quiet night. I lower myself to the curb and close my eyes in silent appreciation of this moonlight sonata.

Saturday when Kaitlin arrives for our date, we stroll through a downtown redolent with the smells of summer. We walk, we talk, and a block away from the swirling black waters of the Cape Fear River and amid the thrum of nightlife, we dine. I like that I can now order wine, so as we settle into our sidewalk table, I request a bottle. It is quickly brought for me to taste, and, pronouncing it good, glasses are poured, and we toast.

"To our first date," I say, raising up the wine.

We drink. The bread comes. We eat. The salads arrive. We eat. And when the seafood lands, we eat, refilling our wine glasses all the while.

"The check, sir," the waiter says, presenting the billfold. And as I count out several twenties, I ignore the great sum spent, telling myself I'm buying happiness.

On our way out, I pause in the door's threshold and mention a nearby coffee shop, adding that it's poetry slam night.

"Let's go!" she enthuses.

So along Front Street, we squeeze between bodies swaying down the avenue in summer intoxication. Clusters of pedestrians form moving walls along the sidewalk, and Kaitlin and I must dodge from one side to another, stepping off the curb and then back on as we go. When we enter the coffeehouse, Kaitlin reserves a table while I order. Then I sit, as a patron reads poetry from the small stage. This young poet muses about love, and although I recognize his meaning, I am glad that it is not something I have written. When he nears the end, his voice crescendos and feedback squeals out from the speakers, deafening me. Then the young poet gives a slight bow to say that he is done. Kaitlin and I smile politely, and we clap. Another poet takes the stage. She reads a poem where she was gifted a dead father for Christmas, and it is sad. Sort of. She steps down. We clap. Another takes her place. I refill our coffees.

Later as we walk back to my house, our conversation carries us along. I tell her about Ana; she talks about Ray, her former boyfriend. I tell her I come from a small town; she says that she does, too. And so it goes, while the moon rises in the east and glides overhead. I stray from any talk about my hemophilia or HIV. There is no handbook for people with HIV, and there are no rules for how I should date, but I know that this, our first date is not the one for such a serious topic. I fear my HIV would ruin any hope I have with Kaitlin.

On my front stoop, the sound of our voices in the night lulls me into a good feeling, and I want us to linger there forever, but eventually Kaitlin stirs.

"I should go," she says. The coffee has worn off, and the date has come to its inevitable end.

"You should have let me pick you up like a real gentleman," I say as we approach her car.

"It doesn't matter. I don't mind driving, and you were closer to downtown."

We hug. Then I feel it: the drawing closer. And we kiss. And it's so uncomplicated, so simple. Before she leaves, we lean in again, breaking apart slowly.

"We should do this again," she says. "Call me."

"Count on it."

After her car disappears, I lock the front door, climb the steps, and crawl outside my window to watch a night as bright as silver day. The stars shine overhead, and the downtown river pulls down the crescent moon. I stretch out and trace constellations on this twinkling canvas, lining out Perseus, Pegasus, and Ursa Minor.

Kaitlin and I share a string of several nights together, all reminiscent of our first date: a walk downtown; a meal; wine; coffee; and a few heavy kisses as my fan whirs beside us laid out on my mattress. I do not push things beyond the roaming of hands, and Kaitlin always leaves before passion overrides reason, at least until a night, two weeks later.

Kaitlin and I have eaten dinner, watched a movie, and we now recline on my mattress reading. I have Flaubert, she Plath. It is late, and Kaitlin stretches her arms out and yawns, letting her book rest in her lap.

"Tired?" I ask.

"Very," she says as she lies back.

I close my book. She puts her head against my chest. The night rustles with kisses and movement.

"Should I go home, tonight?" she asks. "I know it's not that far, but . . . well . . ." She looks to me, and I realize that the time has come for me to tell. We kiss again, and my heart tenses.

So I begin: "When I was a little boy about ten . . ."

When I finish, Kaitlin huddles with her knees between her arms, staring at nothing. It is a moment one could breathe a life between. The night paints us in shadow and mystery and sorrow. When Kaitlin cries, she buries her face in the hollow of my chest, and I hold her and let the darkness fall around us.

I glance around the room and notice Kaitlin's book of poems still open beside her. It was this, I think, she was reading before her life changed. When she falls asleep, I get up quietly and shut my door, turn the fan on low, and pull a sheet over us. I rest my arm across her and lie against her. However, I cannot sleep. Outside, the full moon paints a silver silhouette of the elm tree against my blue wall. It moves ever so slightly as the hours go by and as the fan whirs wind over my sad heart.

In the morning, the shaking bed wakes me and I blink open my eyes and see Kaitlin gathering her things. I kick off the covers, and Kaitlin looks over to me.

"I'm going home," she says. "I can't sleep anymore."

"Okay." I prop myself up in bed, hold the pillow between my arms as if it is her. "Will I see you again?"

"Yes. Don't be silly." She clasps her purse shut. Zips her bookbag.

"Okay. When?"

"I don't know. I need some time, okay. I can't talk right now. There's too much in my head." She stoops to kiss me good-bye—a light peck on my cheek—and suddenly, I am alone in the world again.

I cannot sleep, so I pull myself up and make coffee, thinking of what I should do on my day off. It already feeling somehow spoiled, I try to slug through: a few hours at the coin laundry, another hour divided between lunch and grocery shopping, and several long minutes edging my way through a slow river of traffic. The sun crests the midway point as morning drops into afternoon. I visit the tobacco shop, purchase a cigar, and carry this to a patch of sand overlooking the waterway channel at Wrightsville Beach. White gulls swoop above the water, diving occasionally, and a few vessels motor by, their flags whipping in the coastal breeze and their small carriage sailing underneath the drawbridge. I clip the cigar's end, light it, breathe in, and taste. The yellow smoke puffs in an ocean of sea-blue sky.

For several days, Kaitlin doesn't call. My heart beats uneasily, nettled by unhappiness. But then one afternoon, there is a knock at my door, and, when I open it, she is there.

"I think I just needed time," she says. "I needed to think clearly about this, and I couldn't have you in the way."

"And what does this mean?" I brace myself against the doorknob gripped in my palm.

"I like you." My heart races. "And I think I'd like to work through this. But . . ." My heart slows. "After my last relationship, I felt so used there, and I don't want to feel like that again. I didn't feel like a person. So, already you can see I'm not a big fan of sex."

I clench the doorknob, then release. "I can understand that. We can leave sex off the table for awhile."

"Well, I'm not sure I'm gonna want to for a very long time really. I just wanted to be clear on that upfront."

"Oh. Okay. I see."

"Well really, and more importantly, my abstinence isn't related to . . . well . . . you know. . . . Because it's not. It's a decision I was already working towards." She comes toward me and we hug. "So do you think we can give this a shot?"

I pause, think. "It's definitely worth a shot."

And we are back together as before. We listen to albums and, later that night, we climb underneath my covers, which soon rustle with kisses and heavy petting.

"Is this okay?" I ask as I slide my hand into her panties.

"Yes," she breathes out. "This is great. I want you to." She leans back and nudges my hand lower; then she places her hand in my boxers, and we please one another as we can. A thought crosses my mind whether, without HIV, we'd be having sex, but I squash it and let desire take over, and soon, this quenched, we cuddle close: her chestnut hair tickling my nose while I kiss her shoulder and the nape of her neck.

"I love you," I whisper into her ear.

"What?" she asks, turning her face toward me.

"I said, 'I love you.'"

"Oh . . ." She rests a hand against my face. "I love you, too."

She nestles close. She holds me. I hold her. We pet. We tremble. We sleep.

THE PINE CONE DID IT

September 1993. I pedal through dusk, my bike gliding swiftly along the campus's flat sidewalk. Crickets chirp. Cicadas sing. The fall wind blows and puffs up my loose-fitting shirt. And the fading sun makes silhouettes of trees whose outlines I steer over as I coast. The evening sunbeams flicker through the longleaf pines as a strobe light, and I squint when my eyes water, loosening my grip on the handlebars to swipe a hand over my eyes; and when I can see again, it is too late. My front tire jams into a pine cone the size of my forearm. The wheel locks at ninety degrees and the bike jerks to a stop, throwing me from the seat. I fly over my handlebars and yell in pain when my right foot lodges between the wheel's spokes and twists my knee.

My body pounds on the ground, and the concussive force thrusts a gasp of air from my lungs and flattens my round heart against a hard mat of earth. Then for a moment, the world softens as if in a dream: the swaying trees and the freshly cut grass are chimeras of green, and the autumn air drifts with the perfume of fall wildflowers. I gulp a tentative breath. My heart fills again with blood and returns to beating. Then the pain comes piercing and unrelenting as if slivers of metal are stabbing at my knee from the inside out. I rest against my elbows, catch my breath, and slide myself backwards along the grass to dislodge my foot, still anchored to the bike tire,

83

and as it drops to listlessly rest upon the ground, an intense agony rises from my knee joint. Wrenching my mouth in anguish at the great pain, I labor to breathe as I cup my hands against my knee and feel the swelling. The skin stretches tight against my jeans and presses at the seams, the bloom of swelling restrained only by my patella—a cap upon a boiling radiator of blood.

Turning onto my stomach, I place my palms into damp grass and attempt to lift myself, but a fiery spasm wracks my body, and I grit my teeth and practice slow breaths again. When I regain myself, I muster all my mettle to endure pain and push off from the ground with my arms. It is a great and fierce thrust that lifts me and lets me hoist myself up, where I shift my weight to my left leg to lessen the pain in the injured right one. But still the hurt rages. I bite my tongue and displace the pain to the roll of tasteless skin now gripped between my teeth.

I hobble toward my bike and place a hand upon the frame and ease my injured leg over the seat as if slowly mounting a saddle, and when it dangles above the ground, I push forward with tentative kicks. The wheels move. My leg cries out. I clamp my teeth into my tongue. A whistle of painful air leaks out of the corners of my mouth. I kick again.

When I arrive at my suite, I pull myself up to the second landing and drag my leg through the suite's corridor using the furniture and walls as balances, and then I drop onto my bed, gripping both hands around my kneecap and crying out in pain. I rock back and forth; tears spill onto my shirt; and with my hands still locked around my joint, I try to summon those magical potions from my childhood. *Abracadabra. Make it go away. Abracadabra. Make it go away.* But it does not work.

I phone Kaitlin, who arrives and quickly gets the Vicodin that most hemophiliacs keep handy. Then I show her my knee: the kneecap lost in a globe of expanding flesh. Her hazel eyes widen and then start to water.

"Are you going to be okay?" she asks, marveling at my knee's size.

"Yes. But I need to go to the emergency room, and I need you to drive me there. Get Sean to help. He should be in his room."

She hurries away in silence and from the hallway I hear her fist laying into Sean's wooden door. "Wake up," she yells. "We need your help."

I hear his door fling open and then they return to my room.

"Holy shit," Sean exclaims when I exhibit my knee.

"You gotta help me get to the emergency room."

"Holy shit," he repeats.

He leans down toward the bed, and I shift so that I can reach around his stout neck. "Okay. Put your arms around me." And when he raises me, I pretend that the pain is not real but comes from a phantom limb, one severed from my body long ago. My breath is heavy and winded.

"Go easy," I breathe out. "We have to go slow."

"Okay, okay."

Sean eases me down the stairway and out to the curb while Kaitlin goes for the car, and when she pulls around, I collapse into the backseat, inhaling heavy sucks of dust and heat and letting my knee calm.

At the emergency room, Kaitlin retrieves a wheelchair, adjusts the leg rest, and rolls me into the lobby. We hurry past a woman comforting her sick child, a man cradling his hand in bloody gauze, a lady bent double in stomach pain. At the check-in window, the lady takes my information and my insurance card.

"Blue Cross and Blue Shield?" she asks.

"Yes."

"And you live on the UNCW campus?"

"Yes."

"Any medical conditions?"

"Yes. Hemophilia."

She types. "Anything else?"

"Umm . . ." I pause. I lean in and whisper: "I'm also HIV positive."

"Okay, then. HIV positive," she repeats, typing. "You can have a seat and the specialist will see you momentarily." She points to the lobby where Sean already waits, so Kaitlin and I join him. Kaitlin taps her foot, twists her hands round; Sean shifts in his seat; and I rub my hands on my knee to soothe its pain.

"A pine cone?" Sean questions after I've related the story of my accident. "Jesus Christ, man. How fuckin' big was this thing?"

"Huge, man. Monstrously big."

"Damn. I think I'd go with another story like a raccoon or a deer jumped in front of you. A pine cone just sounds kind of lame. Nobody flips over their handlebars because of a lousy pine cone."

In an hour, a nurse appears, calls my name, and carts me away. She leads me through a succession of double doors that open into a larger room where nurses swarm and where doctors hover near a central desk. They scribble onto charts and rapidly dial numbers on phones the size of mission control centers.

"Do you want me to help you onto the bed?" the nurse offers as we sidle next to one, but afraid to move, I decline. "Well, you should probably remove your pants so that the doctor can look at you," she suggests, tossing me a backless gown with a faded blue flower print dyed on it.

I change, gritting my teeth, and soon lower myself back into the chair where I wait. The clock's hands click off circles. When a sudden pain shoots from my knee, I throw my head back and dream of cutting it off at midthigh and imagine the happiness and relief such an act would bring. *Abracadabra. Make it go away.* My knee is plump, and it feels as if it may split my thin skin in a shower of red, bloody pulp. I close my eyes and try to sleep, but cannot. The clock continues to tick time.

When the young doctor enters, he immediately asks me questions about my HIV and my hemophilia. He wants numbers, figures he can turn over in his scientific mind, so I provide the answers. His team stands behind him, jotting notes and nodding their heads as I explain my situation. When I've run out of things to say and when the young doctor has run out of questions to ask, he adjusts his spectacles along his thin nose and runs a slender hand through a receding hairline, swiping at a tassel of blonde hair. Then he washes his hands and places their cold, clean palms to my joint. I flinch.

"Tender, huh?"

"Extremely painful is more like it."

He feels around some more. "You need your factor," he declares. "I already checked with the hospital pharmacy, and it will take several hours to get here. They don't keep it stocked and will have to order it from another hospital. I wondered, however, if you have any with you?"

"No. But I could get my girlfriend to get me some. It'll probably arrive faster."

He gives a little laugh, a small wind pushing out his lips. "I think that's probably a reasonable assessment. That's fine by me. The nurse can help you infuse." He makes notes in his folder. "So that takes care of the first order of business. Second is the X-ray. We should make sure there's nothing going on in there beyond a bleed. I'll set that up. And third, we should aspirate. Your swelling is severe, and it needs alleviating. Have you had an aspiration before?"

"Yes. When I was little, it was done on both knees. Several times."

"So good. This is old hat to you. You know we're going to insert a needle into the joint and drain as much fluid as we can."

"I know it's going to hurt like hell."

He laughs out again. "Well, we'll give you a local anesthetic to help out, but, yes, with swelling like that it probably is going to hurt some. I won't lie to you there."

I fidget my hands upon my knee, feel pangs of throbbing pulses twitch within and realize that more pain is being prescribed. The doctor leaves and the nurse comes in with water and another Vicodin that I swallow.

"That should help you out," she says, as I pass the empty container back to her.

Then the nurse sends Kaitlin to me, and after explaining the situation, she agrees to drive to campus for my factor.

"But I still can't believe they don't have it here," she grumbles, taking down the list of supplies I call out. "Isn't this a hospital?"

"Well, they weren't prepared for me. I'm just special that way."

When Kaitlin leaves, an orderly wheels me to X-ray, where the heavy machine aims at my knee, clicks, and sends invisible beams of radiation into a mass of bleeding tissue. By now, the pain has eased a bit, but I still bite my tongue as I am helped back into my chair and returned to the emergency room. When Kaitlin arrives with my factor, I mix the bottles, and the nurse infuses me, fortifying me with my clotting agent. Then later as the room's clock approaches midnight, the young doctor and his team return.

"Ah, I see we have good timing," the young doctor says. "You're all factored up and ready to go." He presses my X-ray to the light-box and considers it with a lone finger resting upon his bottom lip. "The good news is that your knee looks fine. It's just a severe hematoma. The bad news is, of course, that we are still going on with the aspiration."

He and his team move me into another, more private room. They lift me onto the table, secure my leg into a stirrup, and then begin yanking on their gloves as needles and syringes are spread out along a tray rolled close by. An attendant swabs me with a sterilization fluid the color of blood, and I watch as it runs from my kneecap, much as the cherry syrup glazed atop an ice-cream sundae. When they shift my knee around for a better angle, pain jerks me; my breath quickens, and my palms sweat.

"I'm going to inject a numbing solution into your joint," the doctor explains while holding the needle above my flesh, "but given the amount of swelling it may only do so much good." He leans over and punctures my knee underneath the patella. I wring my hands together, avert my eyes, and brace against the pain that yanks a cry from my throat.

"Hold his leg still," the doctor commands, and a volley of hands straps me down. I thrash and slam my fists against the bed while the doctor coaxes, telling me to hold on, it'll all be over soon. Then, momentarily, the seething hurt eases and my tears dry up as the doctor waits for the anesthetic to take effect. I grow anxious, anticipating the next needle, which is twice as long as the first one.

"Oh, Jesus," I call out.

"Okay. Hold still." He looks to his team. "Hold him tight." They get into position. The needle comes at me. And this time, it is worse. Pain blazes as the needle jabs into my joint, and when I close my eyes, I see thickets of red and black. My body becomes fluent in pain: rasping breath, trembling hands, thrashing head. Even my heart is a compartment with a burr of hurt lodged within. When I clear for a moment, I see the doctor pulling on the syringe's plunger and sucking fluid into it, as if bleeding nectar from a ripe fruit.

When the doctor says he is done, I lift myself to view my poached knee—a red, unpulped mass. The attendants apply gauze padding and begin to encase my leg in a cast. The modern-day bloodletting has ended.

The nurse comes to me with water and another Vicodin for later while the doctor writes a prescription for more, and then I am passed over to Kaitlin and Sean, who've fallen asleep in the lobby.

"Are you okay?" Kaitlin asks, rising to hug me.

"He doesn't look okay," Sean answers.

"I'll live."

They wheel me into the late night, a world now lit by the hum of electricity and a thumbnail moon. Sean comes with the car, and he and Kaitlin slide me into its backseat, and later lay me to rest in my bed, atop the sheets, and with an ice pack pressed gently on my bandaged knee. My eyes glaze over, and as I give into the darkness, I recognize the weight of Kaitlin's body settling beside me. She kisses my face, tells me it's going to be okay, and eases an arm across my chest. The throbbing pulse in my leg dulls so that sleep, for a time, envelops me.

Near dawn, light strains through my window; the sun is rising. My leg lies unmoving and thrumming with pain. I slowly raise my hands to shift the pillow underneath my head and watch as sunlight paints my room in familiar colors. Kaitlin rouses and runs a hand along my chest. "How are you?" she asks.

"Okay, I guess. But it still hurts like hell."

We lay together until Kaitlin rubs sleep from her eyes and slips out of bed.

"I can run to the pharmacy for your pain meds if you want. They should be open soon."

"Yes. I think I'm going to need it to get through today."

She dresses and leaves. For a time, I lie still watching the red glow of morning. An hour or so later, she returns with the medication and sets it at my bedside along with a bottle of water, and then she ensures that my crutches are close, and asks if I need anything else.

"No. Not for now. I can make it."

"Okay, then," she says. "I hope you don't mind, but I think I'm going back to my dorm to get some rest. I'm glad it's Friday and I don't have any classes."

"No, sure. Go rest."

I sleep. Watch TV. Read. Sleep some more. In the afternoon, Kaitlin returns with food and then after eating, we watch more TV and try to sleep. On Saturday, it is the same. And on Sunday, I attempt a shower. We duct-tape a garbage bag over my cast, and I crutch into the bathroom, biting down the pain as gravity drains blood into my joint. I prop in a plastic lawn chair, and the hot water revives me and soothes an endless ache pumping from my knee.

The following week, I heal. Daily, I treat, my arms becoming pock marks of bruised injection sites. Kaitlin visits my professors and brings my assignments, while she and Sean tag-team the transportation of my meals from the cafeteria. Daily, however, the room closes in upon me. I sleep, read, study, eat, sleep more; in the evening I don the protective garbage bag for my daily shower, and in the night, I sleep again, sometimes with Kaitlin at my side, but not always as she needs her escape from this, from me. By the end of the week with the pain tolerable, I crutch to a table in the campus dining hall. It is good to get out. The leaves are beginning to fall. A handful of sparrows flutter in the treetops and in a sky purpled with whisper-fine streaks striating the horizon.

The next week, I walk a few steps without my crutches, but soon fall back into my bed—the pain shooting through me—but each day I make progress—first to my door, then down the hallway, the bathroom—until eventually I only need my crutches for the long hike to the cafeteria. Two weeks later, the doctor removes my cast, and wraps me in an Ace bandage. In another two weeks, this is removed and he approves a handicap parking pass so that I can return to classes by parking nearby. And so I reenter the classroom, leaning hard against a cane, but glad to be returning to normal.

Several weeks pass. Then on a Tuesday in my philosophy lecture, the professor comes to me before class begins and passes me a sealed letter.

"The administration sent this to me earlier this week," he says. "It's for you."

When I see that it is from the North Carolina Division of Public Health, panic rises. My face whitens.

"Everything okay?" the professor asks.

"Yeah. Sure."

"Okay. Good. This seemed most odd."

He returns to the lectern and addresses the class while I read the letter, which, with words like "urgent" and "pressing importance," demands that I contact the division ASAP. My imagination unreels scenes of disease and horror: I have TB; I require quarantine; my life is ending. Hurriedly, I limp to the handicap parking space, and, back in my room, I call.

"Yes, Mr. Smoak," says a lady on the other end. "I've been trying to get in touch with you but have been unable." Funny, I think. I have a phone and an answering machine, and I have been readily available having been grounded by my injury. "We need to talk," she continues. "How's this afternoon, say three o'clock?"

"Umm . . . Okay."

"Great." And she hangs up before I can ask any questions.

My worry increases. I thrum my hands against my desk. I sharpen my pencil. I open my desk and sharpen all my pencils. Then I test all my pens, discarding those out of ink. I collect all the loose paper clips from my drawer and organize these in a box and then I flip through my notepads and rip out pages that are marked and now useless.

When the lady from the Health Division arrives at my door at three o'clock, she is dressed in a navy-blue sports coat with brass buttons, and she chokes my room with perfume as she enters. Making herself comfortable at my desk, she reminds me of an oversized gourd, like the ones my grandfather hung for spring martins to nest in. She fishes out a file from her leather briefcase.

"I'm Margaret O'Delle," she says, crossing her legs while I recline on my bed, festering with curiosity and concern.

I offer her soda, coffee, or crackers, but she declines.

"It seems you've somehow slipped through our system. You are HIV positive, correct?" She thumbs through her folder, rifles out a form.

"Excuse me?"

"It has come to our attention that you are an HIV-positive male living in New Hanover County. You were recently admitted to the ER, I believe."

"I suppose."

"Well . . . You must understand the extreme threat this virus has caused, and this just lets us know that all precautions are being taken with persons such as yourself." I smile feebly. "So, Mr. Smoak. Have you had any sexual partners?"

"What?"

"Any sexual partners?"

I feel violated. My insides stew. I clench my fists together and squeeze the knuckles white. I am now the enemy.

"Have you had any sexual partners?" she repeats, her steel face revealing no emotion.

"I'm not sure."

"Either you have or you haven't had sexual relations."

"I haven't then."

She taps her pen upon my desk. "I don't believe you," she says, furrowing her eyes on a taped-up photo of Kaitlin. In the silence between us, I hear her steady breathing.

"You asked if I'd had any sexual partners, and I'm saying that I haven't."

"Mr. Smoak, what you don't understand is that we have to follow the names of any partners you've had and ensure that they're receiving the proper care and attention."

"Bullshit. You want to ensure that I haven't infected them."

She folds her hands across her lap and lets out an offended gasp of air. "Calm down, Mr. Smoak. I don't doubt your good intentions, but this is state law, and it can have serious consequences should you refuse."

"I'm not refusing. I simply don't have any sexual partners to offer up to you. Actually, I'm one of those rare breeds that is saving myself for marriage."

"Are you involved in any relationships now, Mr. Smoak?"

"The only relationship I have is with my studies," I retort, drawing up and limping to fling open my door. "I think you should leave. This is over."

"It's mandatory state policy to follow through these things," she says, gathering her things and shoving a blast of air from her mouth.

"Here's what I think of state policy," I say, giving her the finger.

She scurries by, shouts: "I'll be in touch! This isn't over!"

And then she is gone. And I'm on the phone, trying to raise my dad at the Goldsboro plant where he now works. They page him. He picks up.

"Dad," I say. "Dad, oh, I don't know what I've done."

"Calm down, Son. Just calm down and tell me what happened." So I tell.

"What?" he asks when I finish. There is the sound of his angry breath. "Goddammit," he says. "God fucking dammit. If that ain't the shittiest, vilest thing this goddamn state of North Carolina has ever done." He pauses. His anger travels the BellSouth lines to me. I understand him. "I can't believe this shit," he says. "Do you have her number, Son?"

"Yes."

"Give it to me."

I don't ask why? what for? I read the number aloud.

"You've done nothing wrong here. You hear me, Son? You've done nothing wrong. Do you understand me?"

"Yes."

"Okay. I'm gonna call and give somebody a piece of my mind."

When he hangs up, I curl onto my bed, wondering how much more I can take. I don't even get up to put on music, sometimes my only solace. I am alone, singled out, an island again. I just fold into myself, sleep, and only later wake when Kaitlin comes by to check on me.

"I can't believe they did that," she says, sitting on the edge of my bed, listening to my story.

"Me either."

"So, you didn't give me up, did you?" Kaitlin jokes, throwing her arms around me and showering me with kisses. "My hero," she says with more playful kisses. "Oh, it's like in the movies. Are we gonna have to run away? Hop trains? Fake our passports?" She falls against me in an exaggerated swoon and whispers into my ear—"My hero. My hero."

At home after the Thanksgiving holiday, my family and I circle the Sunday dinner table as Mom lays out the fried chicken and mashed potatoes with sides of butter beans, corn, and biscuits. We eat. But it's not long before Dad starts in again against the state:

"Shittiest thing I've ever heard of. Shitty, shitty, shitty," he says.

"Shelby, not at the Sunday table," Mom warns.

"It's just shitty. That's all there is to it. Shitty." He bites into the fried chicken, tearing meat, chewing angrily. Then he points to me with his chicken leg. "Son, I hope you've learned a lesson. Time you sign your records over to some other hospital besides Chapel Hill, see what happens? Those other hospitals don't know you. They just see you as a number and then they report it. One thing your mom and I have learned all these years is to keep our mouths shut and to keep as few people—doctors, hospitals, and whoever—from finding out. People can be mean and thoughtless when it comes to some things, especially when it comes to things about you." Dad lays the leg on his plate, forks his green beans. "I know Chapel Hill's not close for you, but I swear to God you gotta make that drive, no matter how."

"But it was an emergency," Mom interjects.

"I don't care. He should have just kept his mouth shut and not said anything about anything else. If too many people find out about you . . ." He looks to me. "If too many know, I can't even say what will happen when you graduate and start looking for a job. And I know. I see it every day at the plant." He pauses. "Every day there's discrimination. Every goddamn day."

The room stills. Only the sound of our eating fills the silence.

LUNGS

January 1994. I drive to my appointment at the Hemophilia Center and marvel at the piles of snow along I-40. As I swish through thawed patches of slushy roadway, melting winter surrounds me: the sun softens the frozen ground with its feeble heat; the wind loosens powder from the barren trees; and the winter birds caw above the white earth, quieting only when they light in frigid puddles for a drink.

At the clinic, we go through the familiar motions.

"Today," Dr. Trum then says, removing the tongue depressor from my mouth and bringing my visit to a conclusion, "I think it best to begin some preventative therapies." He discards the depressor, sits in his chair, looks back to me. "Since your numbers are declining, we need to prevent common HIV infections like pneumonia, CMV, and TB. For TB, we'll do an X-ray of your chest and check your blood as well, and for the CMV I've scheduled an appointment with the ophthalmologist where he'll check for floaters and other signs of infection."

"What happens with CMV?"

"While it can cause blindness," he says as I immediately imagine it—all life washed to forever black—"I wouldn't worry too much over that. Not just yet at least." My palms whiten as I lock my fingers together. "Our goal here is to prevent infections, and catch them early before they become uncontrollable. Remember it's the infections that people succumb to and not AIDS itself." He pauses, taps his pen on his notepad. "And when you're finished with the X-ray and eye exam, I want you to return here and the nurse will assist you in your first Pentamidine dose. Now, normally I'd prescribe Septra for you—a pill that you could easily take daily—but since you're allergic to sulfa drugs, I'm going to go about prevention the other way and give you Pentamidine instead. The efficacy of both is pretty comparable. Pentamidine is just a little more inconvenient, as you'll have to come here monthly to receive it." Dr. Trum jots notes in my folder, closes it, clicks his pen, and slips it into his shirt pocket. "So," he says, taking a breath, "that's the plan."

I feel danger approaching. My dropping numbers and these new preventative therapies remind me that I am, as I've always been, dying.

I ride the escalator to the second floor, where the X-ray flashes over my chest, and then I follow the signs to the ophthalmology clinic, where, getting lost along the way, I eventually arrive at the check-in window. Later I grip the arms of a large, vinyl chair while the doctor drizzles dilating drops into my eyes and leaves. In a few moments, I lose focus and squint and shield my eyes from the piercing light, but soon the ceiling tiles' tiny perforations blur into a flat and indistinguishable white. When the doctor returns, he darkens the room and, with his special scope, peers into the depths of my corneas.

"No floaters, today," he announces, as he flips on the overhead lights, returning me to a shockingly bright world.

Shading my eyes with my hand, I feel my way along the walls, shuffling back to the hemophilia clinic, where, after my sight returns, I follow a frumpy nurse named Sheila. As we travel the hospital's bright corridor, my mind turns and my breath labors in fearful anticipation of the Pentamidine treatment. The nurse unlocks an isolated door squeezed in at the end of a long hallway, and as she begins preparing the medicine, I sink into the room's lone chair, which faces a TV.

"You can turn it on if you want," she says, but I hold up my book. The nurse smiles. "It's always better to read than let that thing rot your brain anyway."

She draws a clear liquid into a syringe, much as I would my factor, and she dispenses this into a chamber that holds the Pentamidine and that connects to a flexible mouthpiece. Extending this to me, I watch the sterile tubing uncoil and end at a machine the size of a small box.

"This nebulizer," the nurse says, "will push air through that tubing and make a mist of the Pentamidine. When I turn this on, just relax and breathe as you normally would. That's all there is to it. A piece of cake." She forces a little smile as she flips on the switch. "Okay. Just breathe. I can't stay in here with you, but I'll be back in about forty-five minutes to check on you. You should be done by then."

"Okay." And she leaves.

A thin mist like flour rain spreads through the tubing and filters into my mouth, my throat, my lungs, leaving a taste like a pasty mouthwash. The book rests in my lap as I stare at the plaster wall and listen to the nebulizer hum, my lungs inflating and deflating, inhaling and exhaling.

In an hour, the nurse returns, apologizing for being late. She turns off the nebulizer, takes the mouthpiece from me, and discards it in the hazardous waste container.

"That's it," she says, rubbing her hands clean with a disinfectant wipe. "You're all done and free to go home. Guess we'll see you in about a month for the next treatment."

"Guess so," I say, gathering my things to leave.

Outside, the melting snow spreads out like dirty-white tree skirts beneath the evergreens. I pull my wool cap over my ears and blow into my hands and, arriving at my truck, watch as my breath fogs the windshield. Along my drive home, the twilight sky purples and then fades into hushed winter blackness. The half-moon struggles to shine before a few stray snow clouds pass over and blanket its light.

I do not stop at the college, but steer across the Cape Fear River toward nowhere, listening to the thrum of my tires against the drawbridge's metal grate and hearing the dark river slushing below me, still and black. I crack my window and the freeze kisses my left check while the bitter wind chills me and whistles through my cab. It is as if it wants to say something but cannot.

I cough and taste the Pentamidine and spit out the open window. And when I cough again, I put a hand to my chest to be sure that it is only a cough and nothing more. My lungs rattle with cold fear, but they do not gurgle with pneumonia. I am safe. For now.

When I pull into Southport, the main street is empty and its dock desolate. I carry my coffee to the pier's end and gaze across the channel to the Bald Head Island lighthouse: a towering shadow underneath a half-mooned sky, a silhouette against a black, outgoing tide. I cup the coffee to my mouth, blow to cool it, and then sit along the dock, letting the cold dark numb me.

As if weighted down with ice floes, the sable river slugs on. Steadily, it slaps the rocks below me with a sound like a low and mournful moan. I breathe in the night and breathe out a cold mist that plumes before me and disappears as fading vapor in the moonlit sky. The winter chills my lungs, chaps my lips, and stings my nose and ears—freezing off all feeling.

EARS

March 1994. Pollen mists through the air. A pinch of green dusts cars, flours the trees, and sifts upon the college lawn, only made airborne again when a strong breeze unsettles it. Allergic to it, my ears are strangled by fluid. I hear the world as if in a large vacuum, and the noise sounds thick and distant, while speech in a crowded room is impossible to discern. Voices have the low cadence of an immutable rumble.

When I phone Chapel Hill, the Hemophilia Center sets up an appointment with an ear, nose, and throat specialist. A week passes. Then, with my clogged ears, my leaky nose, and my watering eyes, I drive through the springtime rain from Wilmington to Chapel Hill to see this ear, nose, and throat specialist. Dr. Cameron whips into the room where I wait (and have been waiting for two hours) and he introduces himself while rooting around my ears, nose, and throat with a funneled penlight. He pushes back his slick-black hair and as he begins to speak, I can tell that Dr. Cameron is all about speed.

"You're clogged up good," he says, reassuring me that I've come to the right place for repair. He squirts a numbing spray into my nostrils and then forces a probe through me so he can view whatever it is he needs to see. "Adenoids," he says, the scope retreating from my nose and leaving my nostril stinging. "Your adenoids are swollen."

"Not good?" I massage my nose stem, wiggling it around to soothe the ache.

"Nope. Not good at all."

The doctor skirts through my chart, grimaces his mouth, and grunts underneath his breath. Then he sighs and addresses me.

"Usually we just take them out, but here," he points to the chart I can't see, "it says you have hemophilia *and* that you're HIV positive. Wow! That's gotta hurt. Are you mild or severe?" he asks, continuing to read.

"Severe," I say, understanding that his question concerns my hemophilia. "The severest," I add. "Less than 1 percent clotting."

"Know what your counts are?"

This I pair with HIV, it being a virus most concerned with numbers and counting. "Low," I say. "The lowest."

"Hmmm," he thinks. "If we go in and remove those adenoids, we risk bleeding *and* we risk infection."

"What are the odds that the fluid in my ear will disappear and that I can hear again?" I laugh halfheartedly.

"Not that good. Maybe by late summer, perhaps fall . . . but the problem there is that it, too, can become infected. We need to get that fluid out of there and keep it out." He wheels a stool to my beside, sliding on it as he rolls toward me. "What do you think about tubes?" I shrug indifferently. "We can pop some tubes in your ears to equalize the pressure and allow your ears to drain. We use it all the time on little kids and it works fine."

"So, why don't you use it on adults?"

"Sometimes we do. But the tubes only last four, five years and usually by adulthood, the problems are more permanent than when you're a kid." He looks to the wall, the clock. "I think it's the best option for you. Whattaya think?"

"How will it work? Will it hurt?" I am uncomfortable at a procedure seldom done on adults.

"Won't hurt a bit. You'll be out to the world under anesthesia. It'll be a day procedure. You'll come in early, get your factor of course, and we'll pop those tubes in, one in each ear. When you wake, we'll monitor you a bit, then you'll go home. You'll need someone to drive you and I don't think

I'd plan anything for the next day because you may still be groggy from the anesthesia, but otherwise, it's a piece of cake."

"Okay, then. Let's do it."

Several weeks later, I arrive at the hospital to have my tubes inserted. As I slip into an operation gown, Dr. Cameron rushes into the room, and he pumps my hand, slaps me on the back, and assures me that it's going to be a cakewalk. "You'll be done before you know it."

When I am laid out on the operation table, my heart palpitates with fear. Not since childhood have I had an operation, and I am nervous. An orderly positions me on the table while a nurse begins the IV drip, which contains my factor as well as the anesthesia.

"Now count back from ten," she advises as I watch the medicine flow through the tubing. I count ten, nine, eight in rapid succession, and she tells me to slow down, that I'm going too fast. I laugh. She laughs. I laugh again, but louder and more silly. I try to count again but keep laughing. My heavy eyes roll in my head as loose marbles, and soon they no longer catch light.

When I come to in the recovery room, I swivel my head around to take in the surroundings and then lazily raise a hand to my ears where I feel gauze packed tight against them. Inside they itch. A nurse notices me and shuffles over to take my blood pressure, my pulse, my temperature.

"The operation went fine," she says. "You'll be hearing again in no time," she adds with a smile.

I nod my head in understanding, return her smile, but when they bring in my mom and she asks questions about my bleeding ears, I start to doubt the surgery's success.

"That's an awful lot of blood," she says, scrunching up her face with concern. "Is he supposed to bleeding like that? You were giving him his factor during the operation, weren't you? Was it not enough?"

"Give it time," Dr. Cameron responds. "It'll heal. Just give him his factor every day for the next five days, and that bleeding will stop. He'll be good as new."

In three weeks when I return for my postoperative checkup, I suspect problems. Despite my constant factoring to stop it, blood still oozes from my left ear canal, and the Q-tip reddens when I gently probe. Additionally, it hurts and I can't hear. I wait to see what the specialist has to say.

The fast man enters, flips through my chart lightning quick.

"How's the recovery going?" he asks.

"Not sure." I point to my left ear. "Still bleeding."

"Let's take a look." He wheels his stool over, shines his probe into my ear, and declares that my tube has been dislodged. "We need to pop one back in there," he announces as he begins giving orders, directing the nurses to gather things together. "Is anybody up here with you today?" he asks, spinning around to me.

"My girlfriend. She's waiting in the lobby." I pitched today's visit to Kaitlin as a day-trip to Chapel Hill, where I'd make a quick stop at Ear, Nose, and Throat, and where we could then have the rest of the afternoon to do as we wished. But now things are changing.

"That's good," Dr. Cameron says. "You may not feel like driving after this. Some patients get a little woozy from the numbing drops I'll have to give you."

"My truck's a manual, though. She can't drive that."

The doctor pauses, the first hesitation I've known him to take. "Well," he resumes, "we can either do it today, or have you come back another time. My thinking is you need to have it done now. We do this kind of thing all the time, so there shouldn't be any complications. So, what do you think?"

"Well . . ." I pause, feeling as if I'm on a game show. "I guess let's go for it. You're the doctor."

"All right, then."

"Is it gonna hurt?" I'm thinking about pain: all the pain of my unordinary life. Pain lingers in my elbow, in my legs, in my ankles. Pain stays in my heart. But I try to keep it out of my head.

"You'll feel a little discomfort," the doctor says. "But that's it." This is the newest catch phrase of the medical profession—"a little discomfort"—and I realize that it's going to hurt like hell. But I want to hear again. "Here's the drops to ease the pain," Dr. Cameron says as he drips them into my ear. They slip down my canal and burn, and sting, and wet my inner ear, but, alas, they do not work. I feel everything.

Dr. Cameron forces a metal spike into my left ear, and I can do nothing to mute my childish cries. I squirm. I squeal. I bite my lips between my teeth and dig my fingernails into the vinyl chair. I fear that Dr. Cameron is going to pierce my eardrum and drive it through my brain, quieting me forever.

"Almost there," he says as my feet kick wildly, my head restrained by a nurse.

"Almost there," he repeats. "Almost, almost." Pain. Pain. "Okayyyy . . . Got it." The sharp, intolerable hurt subsides and is replaced by a dull throb thumping in my head.

"The tube's back in," Dr. Cameron says, sliding off his gloves.

He gives me some more drops—a lot of good they are going to do—and after making another appointment for two weeks later, I am ushered on my way. Dr. Cameron weaves around me, wishes me a good recovery, and exits into another patient's room. And as I leave, I feel woozy, like Dr. Cameron thought I might.

I wobble into the lobby where Kaitlin waits for me.

"What took you so long?" she asks, rising from her chair. "It's almost one o'clock and you've been back there since ten."

I attempt to answer, but the world carousels me. Kaitlin grabs my arm.

"Are you okay?" she asks.

And then my barfing begins.

I totter toward a trash can, and my insides pour into it. When I stop, I waver drunkenly, and I notice that the waiting room audience watches me, perhaps hoping that their visit will go a little better than mine. An elderly lady whispers, "Oh my stars," and I smile to her. I am worse than drunk; I am sick and drunk. Then, as if choreographed, nurses encircle me and I am quickly coddled away in a coronation of white.

"Let's get you in back," one of them says, guiding my arms, and I give into my dizzy lean and allow them to help me.

Away from the waiting area and in the patient room corridor, I stop. "I have to throw up again," I say, and a green pan is shoved to me. Mouth agape, insides rivering out of me, I wretch uncontrollably in the open door of another patient's room. The man's eyes widen as he looks on, and when I have a break, I give him hope. "Yours'll go better," I say before I am pulled down the hall.

The nurses return me to the room I just left. "It's the drops," one of them says, spreading the white paper across the bed. "They've gotten inside his ear."

"Oh, child," the other nurse responds. "I hope not." She looks at her watch as I begin to vomit again. "Gonna be a long day if you're right."

I lean up to catch my breath and regain my senses, but everything continues to spin, so I tilt my head back toward the green pan the nurse holds. She yells to another nurse. "I need a clean one. This one's filling up." I rest, hurl again, rest, hurl, rest, hurl.

Soon the nurses have an assembly line set up for my barfing. Nurse 1 passes a clean pan to Nurse 2 who holds this underneath my vomit. Nurse 2 then hands her full pan to Nurse 3 who disappears and returns with another green pan that she gives to Nurse 1. This continues while my stomach muscles grow taut. I feel as if I've been doing crunches for half an hour, as if I am ribbing my stomach like those Bowflex men on the commercials. My head dizzies and my mouth tastes like regurgitation, while my insides spill and splash into that little green pan Nurse 2 holds. Oh, I am sick.

At six, the nurse assembly line slows, for I have slowed. I rest between bouts, while the nurses dally around me, consult their watches, and hold onto their pans. Dr. Cameron presses into my room. He gazes at the clock, taps his foot. Nearby, Kaitlin flips through a magazine. The hallway outside has quieted; the rustle of charts and the rush of nurses is replaced by the calm of an ending workday. I am the last patient.

"What time are you being picked up?" Dr. Cameron asks Kaitlin.

"My parents should be here within the hour," she answers. "They live just outside of Raleigh." Understanding that I won't be able to drive until the drops evaporate from my inner ear—which may take several more hours—Kaitlin has called for a ride. She is to drive her parents' car, while her father will steer my manual behind us. It seems we thought of calling my parents, who live two hours away, but I hardly remember. I have not been any help in the planning of my evacuation.

Dr. Cameron looks around the office, then to the clock. "Well, we're almost done here, and this building's about to be locked tight for the night." Dr. Cameron fires quick glances from Kaitlin to me to a nurse. "We're going to shuttle you to the main hospital, where you can wait for your ride and where you'll be closer to help should anything worsen." I understand that I am about to be moved. I understand, too, that Dr. Cameron fails to specify who is to help me should I worsen, but, as if reading my thoughts, he adds, "But that's not going to happen. You'll be fine as soon as those drops dry up." He darts his eyes to me, to Kaitlin, and then to his pit-crew nurses. "Is he ready to be moved?"

"That suppository ain't done much good. He's still throwing up every fifteen to twenty minutes," Nurse 2 says.

"Let's sit him up. See how he does," Nurse 1 advises.

They talk of me in the third person as if I don't exist. I let them. Exhausted from my upchuck workout, I don't care.

"Time to try and sit up," Nurse 2 coaxes as she places her green pan on the nearby sink.

I sling my feet over the bed's edge, right my head. Everything spins. A pan appears before me, and I gag over it. The roll of water in its corner tells me that it has been cleaned for reuse, that I have been spitting up in this one earlier. Stomach clenched, muscles ribbed, liquid comes up, and then I am done. Nurse 3 rolls a wheelchair into the room, and I try to remain vertical, yet the world seesaws around me. I huff an unproductive nauseous gag. Then helped into the chair, I am pushed to the elevator, down, and out the front door while Kaitlin follows and carries our things.

Outside, the sky is a soft purple and a spring zephyr cools my hot face, reminding me of the summer nights I spent sitting outside with Dad, but this vague nostalgic memory fades as my wheelchair and I are hoisted into the shuttle and I throw up once more. Two passengers move toward the rear, away from me.

Nurse 1 and 2 unload me in front of the main hospital near the smokers, and they wish me the best before leaving. "You're gonna be jus' fine," Nurse 1 says. "I'd stay but I don't have a babysitter for my boy," Nurse 2 adds. And then they wave good-bye from the shuttle window.

Beside me, Kaitlin anxiously watches for our ride. She nestles her chestnut hair behind her ears and turns her head toward me.

"How you feeling?"

"Maybe better," I offer, shrugging my shoulders. "Don't want to call it too early."

"I hope it's over," she says quietly.

She returns her gaze to the road, and I feel a pang of guilt and sadness toss inside me. I know she hates this. I was supposed to have had a quick checkup and—thinking that we'd have the rest of the afternoon to stroll Franklin Street, search for books, and sip coffee before driving back home—Kaitlin had skipped her classes and had ridden with me. Yet this has become the unpredictable hemophiliac's day.

A few minutes pass. Smokers come and go, pretending they don't see the sick boy in the wheelchair. I am a common fixture in this setting. I nod to a lady whose eyes I catch and she blinks back, tugs on her smoke, exhales, looks away. A lone pigeon pecks near her feet and then toddles to another spot, pecks again. I sit full into the chair and begin to feel as if my strength is returning. My stomach is quieting, my vision stabilizing.

As we wait and watch the patients being loaded and unloaded into passing vehicles and as my thoughts drift and recount the day, a silver Porsche whips through the drive and stops. Appearing oversized in his tiny toy car, Dr. Cameron half stands and half sits as he draws my attention with the back-and-forth jerk of his waving hand. He yells out over the engine's roar.

"Feeling better?"

I nod my head yes.

"Just a matter of time now. Those ear drops will soon be evaporated and you'll be just fine."

His motor roars. I nod yes again.

Dr. Cameron lowers himself back into the driver's seat and speeds away, giving me a backwards wave. The powerful rev of his polished car and its pristine engine is muffled in my blood-clogged ear.

"Jerk," Kaitlin whispers. "What an asshole. Don't go back to see him," she says.

"I won't."

The sky darkens, and cars motor by our silent thoughts as the evening cools around us. I watch as a woman swaddled in hospital sheets is wheeled out and packed into her car while her newborn infant sleeps in its child seat. I smile for a moment.

"There he is," Kaitlin announces, breaking our soundless pass of time.

A red Chrysler pulls near us, and Kaitlin's father steps out. I notice another man driving.

"Sorry," her father says. "Raleigh traffic was horrible. I've never seen anything like it."

"Thanks for coming," I offer, feeling terrible at the situation I've gotten him and his daughter into. I offer to drive, but her father takes my keys, asks me where I parked. I don't argue.

"Your uncle George is going to drive you guys home."

"Okay," Kaitlin says. They hug and then her father hurries away.

Kaitlin and I get into the Chrysler with her uncle and we leave, the sky now growing stars.

"That must have been some day," her uncle says over the quiet motor's hum. "Some day," he repeats in a faint whisper.

"Yeah," Kaitlin answers back. "It was that, to say the least."

Kaitlin rests her head full into the seat and stares straight ahead as I recline in the back, feeling something more than that seat divide between us. The vomiting over and the world no longer spinning, my ear reminds me of its pain. I recall the spike inside me and the procedure to heal me. The left stings and itches, and I still cannot hear for all the blood sloshing inside it. I palm the gauze against it, but the constant ache persists. The pain out of my reach, I leave my ear alone, for I understand something about being unable to touch the thing that hurts.

YACHTS

May 1994. As college graduations go, mine is no different: full of fanfare and celebration and the excitement of another rite of passage achieved. I cross the stage—the sun smiling overhead—and accept my B.A. in English. And then my family, Kaitlin, and I lunch at a restaurant overlooking the Wrightsville inlet. Dad and Mom chime their wine glasses and toast me, and later they pass me cards filled with green bills; my life after college begins. As we part, Mom squeezes me and effuses about how proud she is of me; she yanks a tissue from her purse to blow her nose, dry her eyes. And then, Dad hugs me and leans in close and whispers in my ear, while his lanky arms encircle me, "Now all you need is a job with insurance, Son. We can't keep you on there much longer. You're aging out."

"I know, Dad. I know . . . And I'm looking."

He pats me on the back, hugs me again. And then, we part.

The next morning, I scan the want ads, seeking a summer job to tide me over until something more permanent presents itself. Later, I call the Carolina Yacht Club, which needs summer help, and after a short interview, they hire me as a summer cabana boy. After doing some rough calculations based on their offer, I accept and cross my fingers that these wages will pay the bills for my apartment living. Indeed, with rent, utilities, car insurance, and so forth—it's going to be tight.

A series of two-story wooden structures whose length would match a football field and whose width—when considering its several buildings—spans the three blocks from the ocean to the inlet side of the island, the Yacht Club blends in with the surrounding beachfront properties in décor and color: beach gray. Its many rooms—kitchen, bar, showers (indoor and out), changing rooms, dining hall—serve as a haven for club members and their guests. Club members can bronze their skin on the property's private beach; swim in its delineated ocean; lunch over rounds of canasta; dine with cocktails of vermouth; dance beneath a solstice sun long gone down; and, well, simply drink beverages poured heavy with vodka, gin, or bourbon. And of course, there is, occasionally, yachting.

At the club, I become known as "The Help." And I help. Sitting in my small cabana, I fetch Band-Aids for children who've cut themselves on oyster shells or who've received splinters from the club's weathered decks; I answer phone calls about luncheons, bridge tournaments, the bar's hours, the ocean's temperature, the weather forecast, and, sometimes, for those interested in taking a boat out, the wind knots; I sell the monogramed hats, T-shirts, shorts, towels, highball glasses, and beer huggies; and, ranking as my most important duty, I screen members and their guests for admittance to the club.

A lady walks up. She gives me her name, says that she is a guest of Barbara Hightower, and I scan my list.

"I'm sorry, Mrs. Clairedale. I don't see that you're admitted for today."

"Well, I declare. Barbara surely just forget to call me in. I told her I was coming. She just forgot." Mrs. Clairedale lowers her large-eyed sunglasses down the stem of her aquiline nose, secures her blowing bonnet atop her head, and gently strokes my wrist, which rests atop the approved guest list. "Can't I just run out there," she asks, pointing to the ocean, "for a quick ray of sun?" She gives me a flirtatious wink. I look right, left.

"Sure. I don't care. It's all ocean to me."

"Thanks, honey. You're a doll."

Hoisting her bag—heavy with towel, book, and lotion—and with her beach chair flung over her shoulder, she saunters off into the sun.

"Was she approved?" my manager asks from behind me. His rough voice startles me, and I jump slightly as I turn to him. "I don't recognize her. Whose guest is she?"

"The Hightowers', sir. She was on their list."

"Let me see your book." He grabs it from my desk and spins it around to where he can read the names. "Where? I don't see her name."

I lean in and read the names, before eventually lighting my index finger upon one. "Right here," I say. "Mrs. Rubenstein."

"That's not Mrs. Rubenstein! Mrs. Rubenstein is the little old lady that comes here every Wednesday to play bridge. She's the Harrisons' guest. That woman you just let use our facilities is definitely not Mrs. Rubenstein." His face flushes red and his voice quavers angrily. The ocean surf drifts between us. "If you're going to work here, you've got to learn the members' names. You need to know who's who." He pauses, furrows his brows at me. "Got it?"

"Got it," I answer.

He slams the book shut, gazes around the cabana, and points at the T-shirts for sale. "Be sure you refold those shirts," he says. "They look disorderly." I give them a glance, think them fine, but keep this thought to myself.

"Okay," I submit.

Later, work quiets. I watch the sea, listen to the salt wind. The late dawn wind sounds like a whorling breeze and bends the cattails to and fro; the sweet smell of salt teases the air; and the ocean spray dampens my hair and moistens my clothes. A string of gulls streams by and closely hovers above the waves until one dives in and quickly resurfaces with its mouth full. The sun not yet scorching, not yet blazing hot—the outside is breathable and pleasant. But by midafternoon, the sun pelts heat, driving vacationers to the strand. The horizon blurs and is only punctuated by the infrequent white catamaran sails cutting its hazy line.

In my free moments, I read, thieving glances here and there because it's against the rules to do anything unrelated to the job. To hide my book, I flatten it in the long center drawer and open to the introduction. No members roam the wooden deck planks and no children squeeze floatation animals between their tiny arms. With my manager away, I steal time as I can.

The next morning, it rains. Nobody shows, for what good is a wet beach? Gray clouds choke the pewter sky that rumbles with thunder. Lightning flashes send an electric branch of pure light from sky to sea. And in its dim and rainy-blue light, I read more, enjoying such simple pleasures: this storm, this book, this quiet. It is not so bad a living.

When I receive my first paycheck, I take Kaitlin out to dinner. We sit at a table overlooking the long pier that extends past the ocean's breakers, and we sip merlot beneath a burgundy sky that soon falls black and is lit up with pixels of starlight.

"Oh, I love that you now have a job and money," Kaitlin says, licking her tongue over her wine-red lips.

"Here's to being out of college and having money." I raise my glass and let the wine roll in my mouth, savoring something more than just taste.

We order an appetizer, salads, the catch of the day, and finish the meal off with desserts and a few more glasses of red wine, and when dinner is done and the bill paid, we stroll along the shore, removing our shoes and wetting our feet in the surf. A few other couples go by, but mostly it is quiet, which gives me the sense that we are alone, together. For a time, we playfully kick water at one another, but the wine causes us both to lose our balance, and we fall against the sand, laughing out loud and then holding one another as the sea sends us its endless whisper.

"Look. You can see it from here," I say, pointing behind us to the Yacht Club, now shut up and dark but looming there yet as a shadowy box. Kaitlin turns around to see. "I can't say that I love that job, but I sure like its money."

"Me, too," Kaitlin adds. "This has been wonderful. Tonight feels rich." She throws handfuls of sand up into the air as if it were money, and it settles in her hair and mine, and we laugh more. We embrace and kiss and roll around in the sand. We lock fingers, press lips, run our hands along one another.

"Maybe we should go to your apartment," Kaitlin suggests.

"Or maybe we should walk farther down the beach where the dunes are bigger and are easier to hide behind."

I smile. She smiles.

She helps me up from the sand, and we scurry along the coast. And when we arrive near the jetty, we slip behind a towering dune and bury ourselves in its darkness, throwing ourselves upon the ground and loosening our pants and using our hands to please each other. She breathes out a heavy sigh of happiness while waves crash and spew foam in the warm night. And after we have done what we can for each other, we turn on our backs and stare up at the sky above, making romantic guesses at the constellations.

"That's Pleiades," I say.

"Oh, I think that's the loop of Orion's belt," she says, pointing up to the twinkling canvas.

I rub my hand across the smooth skin of her belly, snuggle against her.

"Do you think this is how we'll be for the rest of our lives?"

"I don't know," she says. "Of course, we're still young and all that, but I'd like to think that this is how it could be. That's nice to think about."

"It is."

SUNSET UPON THE HEART

SEPTEMBER 1994. AT THE END OF SUMMER, NEW HANOVER HIGH
School in downtown Wilmington hires me to assist with mentally handicapped students. Dad is happy that I sign insurance forms, Mom that I
have a "real" job. And on that first day, as the students arrive, I stand in the
doorway and shake hands as I am introduced by the classroom teacher, Mrs.
McRae. Those returning from the year before already know the teacher, the
classroom, and the school, but a few are as new to this place as me. They
walk slowly, drop their shy heads low and—often escorted by a mother
who coaxes them into staying—they are left in my care. I take one of their
hands—a student with Down syndrome named James whose easy smile and
full round face reminds me of Louise—and I show him where to stow his
lunch, hang his bookbag, and then sit. I give him a deck of playing cards that
he spreads out upon his desk, setting the cards in straight and even rows.

After the bell rings, the class settles down and we go over the introduc-
tions and classroom rules; then Mrs. McRae doles out change for the math
lesson. I stroll the room and cast glances at their worksheets. Sylvia fumbles
the change in her hand and appears to count it, but cannot. I go to her.

"What is this?" I ask, pointing to a tarnished nickel, laid flat on the desk
in front of her.

"A quarter," she says.

"No, look again."

She examines the coin, raises her head to my eyes. "A quarter," she says again. I lift the coin and hold it in front of her, spinning the nickel between my thumb and index finger, and I ask her to think about it, guess the coin. Sylvia lunges toward it, scrutinizes her eyes against the silver, then leans back. "You have pretty hair," she says, reaching out to touch my head.

"No, no, no." I politely deflect her advancing arm. "We're not talking about hair. We're doing math. Counting money." I pick up a quarter from her stack, hold it flat against my palm. "Now, Sylvia. What is this coin?"

She looks to it, staring blank-eyed. "A quarter."

"Good. Now how much is a quarter worth?"

Sylvia opens both hands, extends her fingers. "Ten cent."

In the neighboring desk, Jason has begun to listen. "No, no, no," he says, fetching a quarter from his pile. He pretends he's Sylvester Stallone— big muscles, big man. "Quarter is twenty-five cents." He fishes one more from his pile, then reaches into Sylvia's stash for another. "Three quarters is Coca-Cola." He slaps his desk table, laughs, and tries to pocket the quarters.

"No," I tell Jason. "That money is for learning, not spending."

"Oh, yeah, yeah . . . Sorry." Jason de-pockets the quarters and grabs his pencil to finish his worksheet while Sylvia watches. Then she reaches for Jason.

"He has pretty hair," she says.

"Get your hands away from me." Jason leaps from his chair, tenses his arms, and squints his eyes. "Don't mess with me," he commands in an unnaturally thick and deep voice.

"All right, all right," I interject. "Nobody's messing with anybody. Get back to work and finish your assignment."

Reluctantly Jason sits while Sylvia, mouth agape, stares vacantly at the shampoo sheen of his black hair.

"Quit looking," he says, separating his desk from hers.

"Quit looking, Sylvia," I say. "You need to do your homework."

"Okay, Mitch."

"No. I'm Shelby."

"You have pretty hair like Mitch from *Baywatch*."

"Sylvia. Do your homework."

Sylvia smiles, lobs her head back in laughter and again tells me how pretty my hair is. "You pretty." I thank her for the compliment, advise her to do her work, and move on to another student.

The classroom soon assumes a familiar schedule: math and language in the mornings; lunch; and job and community skills in the afternoons. And then we all grow anxious for the buses to arrive. In a job like this, there is very little time to sit and rest. I must patrol the classroom and teach standing. A lousy teacher, I understand, would laze at his desk and only occasionally take a turn of the room. So Mrs. McRae and I stroll the room as good teachers should, and consequently my ankles swell, as I find gravity and endless standing other nemeses of the hemophiliac.

At my apartment, my body tired and hurting, my ankle now a bulbous anchor swinging from my spindly leg, I factor. Two weeks ago, I had a similar problem and phoned in sick, and the week before that as well, and now I'm out of sick days and must lose pay; and in addition, it all looks very bad to miss so much work, especially for a new employee, but yet I am injured again and cannot walk without causing further injury. By missing tomorrow, I might actually have the chance to return and miss less later. At least this is the mental back-and-forth I go through before picking up the phone to call my supervisor at home. To explain my string of absences, I relate that I have an old childhood injury that has been flaring up.

"Oh, did you injure yourself playing football? Or soccer? Or something like that?" she inquires, trying to understand my increasing absences.

"No, neither. It's a childhood injury, like I said."

"Oh." And then there's a long pause before the supervisor comes back to me. "Okay, well . . . I guess we'll get a sub. Hope you feel better soon," she says. "The children miss you when you are out."

"And I miss the money," I think to myself.

I place an ice pack on my ankle and fall asleep on the couch until the phone rings. It's Mom wanting to catch up and see how I am doing. "I'm fine," I lie (no reason to get her involved in this). "Good, good. You like the job?" "It's fine, too." And we chat a bit, hang up, and then I try to nap before the phone again rings. It's Kaitlin telling me that she's running late and not to wait dinner on her because she needs another hour or so at the library.

"I'll just grab something on my way," she says.

"Okay."

Deciding it's too late for a nap, I heat some soup, refresh my ice pack, and turn on the TV. I nevertheless fall asleep until Kaitlin knocks on my door, wakes me, and we snuggle ourselves into bed. The light off, the quiet night descends upon us. Kaitlin shifts, turns on her side, on her back, turns back onto her side.

"It's not the same," she whispers.

"What's not the same?"

"Us. This."

I roll over to face her, but she averts my eyes and stares at the ceiling, at nothing while her face is cast in the silver shadow of moonlit dark.

"We used to study together, but now you don't have any studying to do. Plus, you're too tired to even stay awake, or your ankles hurt too much, and so we don't do much of anything. At least not together. We meet and we sleep and sometimes we eat together. It just feels different somehow. Like something's changed."

I sigh. "I'm just adjusting to this job. That's all. It's a lot harder than being a little cabana boy at a yacht club, and it makes me feel pretty awful sometimes. So yes, that's changed. But I can't help it. I'm trying my best."

"Yeah, I know, but you're at work all day and then you're asleep all night and we're hardly talking." She sighs out heavily. "What are we doing?" She looks at me, her cobalt eyes holding steady in the void of night.

"Living, I guess. Gathering our rosebuds while we may."

"Oh, Herrick's no good to us now."

"Yes. I suppose not."

I slip toward her, kissing her cheek and neck, trying to bait her lust. She pulls away and brushes me off.

"Not tonight, okay. I'm not in the mood."

I shuffle back to my side of the bed and lie still as my frustrated desire softens.

"Are we ever going to have sex?" I whisper out.

"Oh, that again."

"Well, are we? We've been dating over a year now."

"I don't know. I told you from the start how I felt."

"Are you afraid of me? Of it? Is that what this abstinence is about? If it is, please just tell me so I can deal with it."

"No," she defends. "That's not it at all. I also made that clear when we started going out."

She rolls onto her side, her back facing me. The moonlight slanting through my blinds crisscrosses our bodies, while outside I hear the soft tread of a neighbor walking her dog and a voice placating, "Good boy. That's a good boy."

Sometime later, I fall asleep.

The next evening, having been home from work and now feeling better, I call Kaitlin and leave a message. I call again and apologize and say that I'll work on spicing things up. And later, I again call, but having heard nothing from Kaitlin, I begin to worry. I try to read for solace, but cannot. Half-hourly, I phone her apartment until, eventually, her roommate answers.

"I'm trying not to get involved," she says, "but Kaitlin's not here and you can't keep calling. I'm sure it's nothing, that she's probably just studying late or something, but seriously, I can't even watch TV for the phone ringing."

"Okay, sorry. Just let her know I've called."

"I did that the first time you left a message."

I pace my carpet, limp around on my stiff ankle. I go outside and sit on the steps overlooking the parking lot, and each time a car pulls in, I try to discern in the dark if it's Kaitlin returning from a late-night study session. But it never is and at two o'clock, I can take it no more. My heart squeezes blood in tight, palsied pumps. I tremble uneasily.

The husk of night shrouds around me and the bright stars pierce light past a hidden moon as I raise my hand and gently knock on Kaitlin's apartment door. The guff of a car comes to me, and I quickly spin round to see if it's Kaitlin, but it is not and the car passes. I knock again, louder. Nothing. I bang again and again so that the metal clapper clamors through the silent darkness, and soon a yellow ebb of light glows from within. The bolt clicks, and when the door opens I feebly smile to Kaitlin's roommate as she sleepily gestures for me to come in. "I'm so sorry," I say. "I'm so sorry." Without saying a word, the roommate relocks the door and ambles off to her bedroom at the hallway's end. I am left alone in the dark apartment.

I fumble my way toward Kaitlin's room, and when I open her door, I search for some sign that may explain her disappearance, but there is none. Her room is as it always is: neat and orderly. I crawl beneath her sheets and wait. Everything falls silent. The faint sniff of her perfume upon the sheets reminds me of her and I ache in a way far different from those pains caused by my hemophilia. I thrum my fingers upon the mattress, toss right and left, fluff up the pillows underneath my head, and when the sun rises and Kaitlin has still not come home, I rummage through her desk, find paper and a pencil, and write a short note, describing as best I can my insufferable night. I tell her that my heart feels skewered, a spit stuck through its center and roasting, but this then seems too much, so I ball it up, force it into my pants pocket and begin again. *Call me,* I write, and then leave.

At my apartment, I brew coffee—extra strong today—and dress for work. Kaitlin calls before I'm off.

"I'm sorry," she says to my sullen hello. "I should have called."

"Where were you?"

"With a friend." There is a long pause. An empty pall settles upon me. Her tone tells me all I need to know. "I know you have to work, but we have to talk. How about tonight? Dinner?"

"What time?" I ask, my voice staying flat, unemotive, and drained of any willingness to appear anything but hurt, dejected, lost. I am numb.

"Five?" Kaitlin offers.

"Okay."

And we hang up. The long night has ended. A new day begins.

Too early for work, I drive to the riverfront park and sit in my cab to think. A barge slugs out to sea and, furrowing the waterway, churns an auburn foam from the murky river. The sky is clouded over and a steady rain begins to pummel down and spill onto the rivertop. It comes heavy and relentless, glazing my windshield. I breathe in, and then a great sorrow comes out of me as the rain, too, cries.

When Kaitlin and I meet, it is early. In the diner, an old man sits alone and sips a cup of coffee, his hand trembling with age. I walk to a window booth where Kaitlin waits, and I shake off the rain from my coat as Kaitlin stands. We hug, then I sit and look outside at the drip of rainwater spilling from the diner's gutters. The waitress comes, and when we order I catch Kaitlin's eyes. She smiles but says nothing. We return to watching the traffic. And later, when our food arrives, I organize my plate, take a few bites, and then fix Kaitlin with a stare.

"Do you love him?" I ask.

"I don't know. It's too early for that." She turns away, pinches at a biscuit.

"But you have feelings for him?"

"Maybe." Kaitlin sips sweet tea. "I still love you."

"But not in the same way?"

"No. My feelings have changed."

I stare out the window to the cars lined up under a sky of rain. Inside, it is quiet. I am quiet. Kaitlin is quiet.

"Is this about my ankles? My ears? My HIV? Is it because I go to the hospital like other people go to the mall?"

"No. Not at all. It has nothing to do with that. It's me."

"Did you sleep with him?" I blurt out. "I have to know."

"Well, no. Of course not. At least not like you think. But, yes, I did stay over there." She says that she is sorry and apologies float from her mouth in a weightless and invisible stream of language. She still wants to be friends. She didn't want it to happen, not like this at least.

"But it did happen."

She turns her eyes away and looks outside. "I guess so," she replies sorrowfully. "It did."

"Then it's over? We're through?"

She sniffles. "I guess so."

With that comment, it is as if my heart has been looted of all its love. When I slide out from the booth, preparing to leave, Kaitlin glances up at me, a loose tear slipping from her eye.

"Why?" I ask.

"I don't know. I don't know. It just happened."

Kaitlin folds her hands over her face and slumps her body forward, and I suddenly miss her terribly. I want to console her and comfort me and pretend that this isn't happening. But I don't. Instead, I shrug my shoulders, shake my head in a gesture of regret and incomprehension, and I leave. *Perhaps this is best,* I think. *We never really consummated the relationship anyway.* Oh, I am hateful in my rationalization. But, no matter how I turn it, it still brings me to tears.

I sink into my couch and watch the rain and then I watch it stop and then I watch the sun begin to peek out. My apartment seeming a cell of sadness, I drive to the beach and push out into the warm fall water as the waves rise above me and swallow me. Even though the sun shines, the sea is full of cold rainwater. I let myself sink below the waterline and imagine what it would be like if I never surfaced.

Not knowing where else to turn but to a friend, I visit Sean, and as I park, I see him reclined in a lawn chair outside his apartment. The sun hangs low in the sky and Sean's chair faces its descent. I walk behind him, smell his cigar.

"She left me," I say to his back and the descending sun.

"Kaitlin?" He exhales smoke from his stout cigar.

"Yes. Kaitlin."

"That's too bad. That's rough." Sean reaches beside him and pulls another chair next to his. "Have a seat, my friend. Watch this sunset with me."

I sit. I look to Sean. He gives me a wink then flicks his cigar toward the darkening sky, directing my gaze. The sun perches on a grove of far-off pines, their greenery washed black into a ragged silhouette horizon line. This dusk, the sun is bulbous in the sky: a giant glowing orb of warmth and light. Then the sun dips; its bottom lip hides behind the evergreens. As it descends from view, the sun projects a thin curve of light over dark pine and paints the pastel sky in shades of supple lavender. A plane has flown across, and its exhaust puffs up as cumulous and pretends to be its own cloud as it colors this baby-purple dusk in its manufactured whiteness.

Sean draws in his cheeks, inhales a shallow taste of cigar. "Gorgeous," he declares. "Absolutely gorgeous."

I agree and nod my head to say so.

"That's what you have to think about, my friend. Kaitlin," Sean says, thumping cigar ash against his metal chair, "is no different than that sunset. With a sunset, for a time you shine in the glory of that beauty. It makes you happy. You feel good. And you're part of it. But then it's gone. It fades and all you're left with is the memory of it. And you know what the hardest part is?" I say that I do not. "The hardest part is realizing you have no control over it. No control at all. You just have to let it be. You have to understand that some sunsets are longer than others." He exhales, breathes in. "And I say that one," he points to the sky, still a faint purple, "is quite a good one. Even grand perhaps."

"Is this *your* metaphor for relationships?"

"Well, not mine completely. Somebody else's ideas translated by yours truly. But that doesn't matter."

We sit quietly for a moment as the night ensues.

"Well, how do you explain the relationships that last, the ones that don't end?" I ask.

"Oh, they end," Sean says, seeming ready for my challenge. "Sadly, everyone eventually ends, and that is their sunset, their purple going black."

"I guess that's true," I allow. I lean back in the chair and make out the feeble light of a few stars. "I think for my next relationship, Sean, I'm going to aim for catching a girl who is like the sun around the middle of June."

"Yeah. That's good. I suppose, then, that my last one was more like a December sun. Short and cold." I give a half-laugh at his humor, then turn back to the evening sky.

We sit mutely for a moment, lost in our separate worlds of thought. I imagine Kaitlin and half wonder if she's with *him* tonight, but the thought is too vivid and painful to consider. I tousle a flip of my hair as, around me, the diamond evening fades into coal night.

THE HANDBOOK TO

DATING WITH HIV

In my apartment, with nothing but the winter's howl outside, I brew endless cups of coffee, prop my feet up on the couch, place a cold compress on their swelling, and I read. I glance up. The light outside darkens and a lone branch brushes against my window in a frigid breeze. Sleet falls and patters against the glass, the rooftop. I draw my blanket around me to keep winter from freezing all of me.

In spring, the crabgrass grows high; the buttercups open and reveal their hidden anthers; and the azaleas bloom in coronations of white, yellow, pink, and red. And although the cold winter is now behind me, it yet lives in my heart.

One evening William calls. He says that he wants to come to the coast and live, so we decide to make a go of it as roommates, and a few weeks later, he moves down. While I'm at work, he searches for a house—one with a sizeable backyard for his dog to run free in—and an afternoon that very same week, as I remove my work shoes and prepare to settle the customary ice pack upon my ankle, William returns, jubilant and talkative.

"I've found one. It's perfect."

We drive to Castle Hayne, a small outskirts community affixed to Wilmington, and we tour a ranch-style brick house whose size is almost equal to that of my parents' home. A large glassed A-frame arch tents over the den area, and the brick house stretches outwards from both sides of this and is trimmed in fresh white. Inside, the owner has rolled out new carpet, painted the walls, and put down new linoleum in the kitchen. I marvel at its newness, at its vastness.

"So how much is he asking?"

"Seven hundred a month," William says. "That's three-fifty a person."

I mull it over. Currently I pay $325 a month for rent, and $25 more for such a large place hardly seems an excessive increase, so I sign the rental agreement. It is only later that I realize the yoke of this house. Costs included in my apartment's rent (the water bill and trash collection, for example) but not budgeted here will soon deplete my paycheck, while the enormity of our summer electric bills (a result of overrunning the air conditioning to keep the house tolerably cool) will leave me slack-jawed and newly attuned to the paucity of my earnings. But these burdens follow. Today, I feel the slight grant of clemency as levity supplants gravity. With the sheets signed and with the keys in hand, I run through the empty house, arms akimbo, all smiles.

The following afternoon, we move our furniture. It does not take long, for we both have very little, so little in fact that even with our things in them, the rooms exude an empty and unlived-in feeling. I fill my room with a bed; a stand of crates that I use as a dresser; a waist-high bookshelf overflowing with novels, read and unread; and the stereo, its two speakers, and several dozen CDs which are stowed in boxes of varying size. In his room, William wrestles a dresser into the corner, and although the top drawer is split and several drawers lack handles, he finds his Goodwill item useful. He lays his mattress atop the carpet and also has a cactus under his window that gives a little life to our place. In our den, we set my old Zenith TV atop a plain table that yaws to the left, and we square a couch against the long wall facing the fireplace. In this couch we are lucky, for it appeared in my apartment's dumpster as William and I were moving out, and needing one, we promptly hoisted it into the back of my truck, and, after some fabric cleaning and repairing its one broken leg (probably the reason for its disposal), the couch has a new home.

As evening approaches, we make grilled cheese sandwiches and then we unscrew the cheap bottle of wine we purchased for our move-in celebration. We sit on our back deck and toast ourselves to happiness. The yard is spacious and lined by a grove of poplars, and a pair of robins twitter in the air and briskly swoop from limb to limb, flitting in front of me before alighting in a dogwood off to the backyard's right. Nearby, William's dog wanders about, sniffing here and there in her new home.

"We should go out tonight and keep on with our celebration," William suggests. "Besides, it might brighten your spirits. How about Lula's? You like that place, don't you?"

"Lula's it is."

In downtown Wilmington, William and I walk the long stone hallway to this underground tavern, a local favorite. Its entrance always reminds me of Poe's "The Cask of Amontillado," and on my way out, if I've had enough beers, I imagine that I can hear the name Fortunato being called out from behind its walls.

Inside, William buys the first round of PBR drafts and we carry the pints to a small table in the rear. William lights a cigarette, pulls heavy on it, gulps his beer, and then lounges against the bar chair.

"When it gets here, it's going to be a good summer," he proclaims.

The first beers go quickly, so I set us up for the second round, spilling foam on the floor as I already totter a bit from the wine and the beer. The alcohol warms and enlivens me and unhinges my tongue.

"This summer," I tell William, "I'm going to find me a girl."

"Good for you. So you're finally over Kaitlin?"

"Oh, yeah. At least I think so."

The crowd packs in and the bar roars with the sound of heavy voices and clinking glass. Smoke reddens my eyes as I drink another pint.

"But, you know, William. It's not easy for me to date. You see, there's no handbook. No *HIV for Dummies* or anything."

"Oh, come on, now. You're just being hard on yourself. I think you've done pretty damn good. This is just a low point."

"No, really it is hard. I'm being serious."

"I know you are. And yes, it's bullshit that you have to deal with this. But I think you've done pretty damn good. Myself, I haven't had a girl in three years. Not since Kelly at least."

"Well, I've created my own dating rules, you know. These are to help out the heterosexual HIV-positive male who's trying to get a girl. There's Rule 1," I explain loudly while tilting back my beer. "Smile and laugh like you are the happiest fuck in the world."

"That's good," William says. "No one wants a sad fuck for a date."

"No, of course not. Who wants to date a sorry old sod? And, even more, who wants to date a sorry old sod with HIV?" For emphasis, I pound my fist upon the table. Then I motion for William to quiet his vociferating agreement. "Now here's Rule 2," I interject. "On your first date, if they ask why you limp, discount it as a sprained ankle. Never, ever mention hemophilia on that first date . . . Too many connections can be made. I think it's just better to make a slight lie about my ankle than to invite anything that might have to do with HIV." I sip my draft. The room blurs in a dim fluorescent haze while the thrum of rowdy chatter hums in my ears.

"Hmm," William says thoughtfully. "That's insightful. Well thought out." He affects an exaggerated contemplative manner by placing his hand beneath his chin in the attitude of Rodin's *Thinker*. "And pray tell, what is Rule 3?"

"Rule 3," I announce. "Reveal your HIV on the third date, and, when the news is dropped, the apocryphal look returned to you in her eyes, immediately relate yourself to drama and call this your one tragic flaw."

"Ah, yes," William says. "The tragic flaw. Your Achilles' heel." He sips his draft. "But why the third date?"

"Well, I'm still doing the research, you understand, but that seems to be the time when things either heat up or run cold. If you wait too long, well, your girl's going to begin to wonder why you haven't made any advances. But if you spill the beans too early, it'll chase her away. Why would she stick around after hearing something like that?"

"She probably wouldn't. At least not any of the girls I've met down here. They seem more interested in a frolic in the ocean." He gulps the last of his draft. "So, are there any more rules?"

"Yes. Rule 4: If you find yourself masturbating excessively, go back to Rule 1."

William laughs heartily and bangs upon the table making our beer glasses dance and my full beer slosh over the side and onto the table. By last call, we have polished off several rounds, and when I swagger out, hearing Poe's victim from behind the stone, it is late and the downtown is spilling out its inebriated patrons. We walk past the restored mansions along Front Street and, passing before the Front Street Inn, find ourselves invited to a party happening on its balcony. We share beers with lively and festive vacationers from Canada before later excusing ourselves and making our way toward home.

"Are you okay to drive?" I ask William as I unlock the door.

He takes my keys from my extended hand.

"Of course. You're the lightweight here. Just close your eyes and you'll be fine."

When I slide into the passenger's seat with William at the wheel, I wonder if we shouldn't take a cab, and though I notice a peculiar look in his eyes, something vague and hazy, he walks straight enough to drive.

A light rain falls and causes the swash of the ride to hum its gentle lullaby. My head lobs to the right, to the left, and several times I detect the car slowing, stopping, then speeding again. I come to for a moment and swivel my head round, noticing a man riding in my truck's bed, getting wet in the light rain.

"Whass that guy doin' here?" I ask William.

"Oh, he needed a ride," he says casually.

"Oh." I think awhile. "Do we know him?"

"No. Just met."

"So he's a . . ."

"Hitchhiker, yep."

My head rolls around for a time, then stills itself.

"Is that safe?" I ask.

"Nope. Not at all. But we're living dangerously tonight. Driving drunk and picking up hitchhikers. Yee-haw!!!"

We stop at a darkened house along the roadside and the man in back jumps out and gives us a wave of thanks before William pulls away and I am lulled back to sleep. William nudges me.

"We're here, you party animal."

Inside, I stumble out of my clothes, slip underneath my sheets, and fall asleep dreaming about the last girl I remember seeing. She was tall and had brown hair and sat at the end of the bar where I could see the butterfly tattoo on her lower back and, sometimes, the thin line of her black lace panties. I watched her throughout the night, shooting casual and unsuspecting glances her way as I talked and sipped my beer. I think of her as my hand does what it can and as I momentarily recall Rule 4.

MY LOLITA

June 1995. Coming upon the Deluxe Café—a favorite coffee-house of mine—I order a regular and I read of young Werther's sorrows. They are not mine, for coffee is making me happy again. Today, I feel the precious balm of solitude; the youthful summer warms my heart and stays off the sadness of my lonesomeness.

When I step to the counter for a refill, I notice the young girl sitting there. Her brown hair is drawn into a bun pierced by sticks that make an X behind her head; her blue eyes sparkle from the reflected light of a mirror hung behind the coffee bar; and when she smiles—a seductive spreading of her red lips that reveals white, unstained teeth—and reaches for the sugar, she nonchalantly brushes her hand against mine, sending a quiver of excitement through me. At this point, she shamelessly stares at me and appears uninterested in the young boy with broad shoulders and a marine haircut who talks to her. I catch her eyes on me again, and it electrifies me. I hop-scotch her eyes as the bartender refills my cup.

"I'm Charlotte," the girl says abruptly, breaking her conversation with the boy and being obvious and forward as she extends her hand.

"Nice to meet you." I shake her hand, a light pumping up and down. "I'm Shelby."

"Shelby." She looks up to the ceiling. "That's such a great name."

"I'm quite fond of it myself."

"What's your last name?" she asks, bending her head low to light a ciga-rette between her lips.

"Smoak," I say, smiling with silent humor. Charlotte looks up before lighting. "Shelby Smoak. That's my name."

"Oh." She chuffs at my joke, takes a drag, exhales over her head, away from me. "A writer's name," she declares. "Do you write?"

"Not really. I have a few poems and I keep a journal."

"That's a start. What do you do?" She is assertive and guides our conver-sation as she edges her chair nearer. "You look like a teacher."

"Well, actually, I am."

She exhales like an actress and shuffles even closer. "Have you seen me before?" Her face is less than a foot away, and I needle my eyes around her faint freckles for recognition.

"I don't think so. But it's likely we've crossed paths somewhere."

"Probably. Wilmington might think it's a big town, but really, it's not. It's a small town with the big town appeal . . . but here," she adds, smiling, blowing smoke over her shoulder, "our paths have definitely crossed."

"So they have."

When her friend begins rousing for the exit, Charlotte grabs the bar-tender's attention and asks for a pen and paper upon which she scribbles her number.

"Call me," she says, extending the paper to me. And when our fingers touch, a thrill shoots through me. "Any time after next week is fine." She stands, extinguishes her smoke, shoves hands in her pockets to straighten their folds, and is gone, winking one last time at the door. I fold the paper neatly in my wallet, as I secretly reach out to her.

The following day during lunch as I pass through the high school courtyard with a few students, us just returned from a morning walk, I hear my name called. I turn and there Charlotte squats in the grass, catching my eye. I tremble. She is a student here.

"Now you recognize me?" she asks, giving me that coquettish smile I recall from the night before.

Life has turned on me yet again. My immediate response is to slink away as my gut reels with the monstrosity of teacher-and-student liaisons. But I cannot leave. Somehow I'm already smitten with the charge of impropriety.

"Ah," I say casually as she shields her eyes from the brilliant sun. "So you go here?"

"For two more days, I do," she counters. "That's why I said call me next week."

"Clever. Very clever."

She lays herself out on the grass while I stand over her in an awkward stance that highlights my towering height above her. I cannot help but wonder how she is sizing me up.

"So will you call?" she asks. "I was sincere."

"If I do call you, you should call me by my real name, Humbert Humbert."

"Haha," she says. "You can't be much older than me."

"And you are?"

"Eighteen."

Eighteen, I think to myself. *That's good. Very good.*

"And how about you?"

"Oh, I'm as old as twenty-two," I answer back. "But I'll soon be twenty-three."

"See there. We're not that far apart in age. In the grand scheme of time, we're practically twins." She flicks a strand of her hair from her face, works her charm.

When the school pours out its students for the summer, I call Charlotte. She is young and beautiful, and I have done nothing but think of her the past week.

"I wondered how long it would take you to phone me," she says flirtatiously. "Only two days since school let out," she says, clucking her tongue. "You must be pretty hard up."

"Oh, I am. And oh so weak."

"So, why don't you come by tomorrow? You can start being my Humbert, then. Mommy will be away at work and Daddy left me oh so long ago," she says sportingly. "It'll just be us."

The next day, I am given a quick tour of her home before we find ourselves in the sitting room where the sun shines brightly on an upright piano that she begins to play. From the moment she strikes that first note, I am stricken with a desire for her. She plays very well, and in the cool shade of her parlor with the ceiling fan blowing upon me, I breathe more freely again. She finishes and turns round to me.

"That's a love song, you know."

"Ah . . . and what is the world to our hearts without love?"

"How poetic." She trifles with her hair, twirls it in her fingers. "So you *are* a writer."

"Not really. Those are somebody else's words. From a book I'm now reading."

We leave to grab a bite to eat downtown. We stroll the riverfront. And later as the afternoon heats, we grab cups of iced coffee and amble carefree back to her place. The azaleas long since having lost their blooms, star jasmine and candytuft flower our walk in yellow and white, and the impatiens are just beginning to open their corollas. In the Wilmington breeze, as the smell of gardenias drifts to me along Market Street, I lose my senses and, despite Rule 3, I speak about my tragic flaw. Charlotte freezes, stunned into immobility.

"But you look fine," she says. "I never would have guessed. I mean you have a little limp, but that's it." We walk on as Charlotte asks questions. "So you're not sick now?"

"No."

She pauses next to a fence and reaches through the lattice, snapping a flower from its vine. She removes its petals and drops them in our path, and when there are none left, she twirls the green stem in her hand.

"I'm glad you told me. I know that must have been difficult . . . Funny, too, I just heard a statistic recently in health class that said our generation will likely meet somehow with HIV before we die. And here you are. Funny, huh? . . . I guess that makes you like Humbert with a twist."

"Oh, yes," I say. "I'm what you might call the modern-day *Lolita*. All sultry, seditious, and now, dangerous!"

She leans toward me for a kiss.

"This is safe, isn't it? Kissing?"

"Yes. Why? Do you feel weird kissing me now?"

"A little. But isn't the idea of a kiss that you don't think about it. That you just enjoy it and let it be."

"That is the idea," I say as we kiss again.

On her porch, Charlotte pumps her feet to keep the swing moving and she hums a little tune, the one she played earlier, and comments that she cannot get it out of her head. And as we talk, the distance between our ages fades and begs to be forgotten. Her words drip honey and her speech is smoother than oil.

"You should kiss me again now," she says with a wanton grin spread upon her beautiful face. "Before Mommy comes home and finds us together."

So I unroll an arm around her and draw us together. Below the waist, I am a sure compass, fixed and pointing.

A few evenings later, we drive out to the sea and swim and splay ourselves upon the shore as the sun fades and casts our lust in twilight's shadow.

"You should come to my party tomorrow night," I say as we lie upon towels, watching the sea spread out before us. "It's for my birthday."

"A birthday? Wow? You are getting to be an old man. And tomorrow you'll be even older."

"So it would seem."

And the next day when Charlotte arrives, the party is in full swing. William and a few of his friends make use of the wide-open space of our new home by tumbling across the sprawl of our carpet. They perform summersaults, head stands, splits, and awkward rolls. "Ten," someone yells out after William takes a dive. "That was definitely a ten." Sean drags a speaker from my room into the den and, refusing to participate in the gymnastics, only puts his beer down to play air guitar to his favorite riffs.

Charlotte finds me on the back porch and kisses me as she wishes happy birthday. "Smell this," she says loudly over my stereo playing in the background. She pulls a gardenia bloom from behind her back. The huge white petals fragrance heavily of summer—a sweet southern scent that can only be described as familiar and natural.

"That's nice."

Charlotte smells the flower again. "I got this for you. I thought you might like it. You can put it in your room or something. It'll smell like that for a couple of days."

I breathe it in again. "It will be better than all that incense I usually burn." I take the gardenia, set it against the deck. "I'll leave it here for now," I tell Charlotte as we stand awkwardly for a few moments.

"Want some beer?" I ask.

Charlotte smirks. "Now you know I'm too young." She flutters her eyelashes in mock-bashfulness as I stand there not knowing how to respond. "Oh, you're so gullible. I'm only kidding. Sure I'll have a beer."

We go inside for the fridge and then return to the porch where it is quieter and where it seems as good a place as any to talk. We sit close. We kiss when few are looking.

"You should show me this place. Why don't you give a little tour?" she requests.

So, we go through all the rooms, each filled with partygoers here and there, and then she asks to see the outside. We go out front, and when turning the corner to the side yard, we grab ourselves together in a bundle of lust. Our figures sway in the moonlight. I press her close to me, and if not for her dark eyes being closed, she would see my hungry eyes. Her little mouth and pale cheeks and hair the color of bourbon are beautiful, and for a moment she yields them to me. They are as little glowing treasures in the stiff and dark night, and I feel as some brute thing thieving them.

She breaks our embrace, stills us, and rights herself by brushing down her shirt and adjusting her undone hair.

"I can't stay much longer," she says.

"So you're leaving?"

"Yes. You didn't think I was going to stay the night, did you? You know I have a curfew."

"You do?"

"No, silly. I have to work early in the morning. That's all. Besides, you should hang out with your friends some."

It crosses my mind that we have pushed things too far, that I have somehow overpowered her. Perhaps my boiling passion has, without my knowing it, become brutish, but Charlotte throws her arms around my neck, lays her soft cheek against me, and in a warm hug whispers, "I do need to go, and I didn't want to start what we couldn't finish. Not here. Not tonight with a party raging around us."

"Well how about dinner? Tomorrow night? I could cook for you."

"Tomorrow's no good. I have plans."

"Plans? What . . . a date?" I tease.

"Perhaps. He's a friend . . . like you." My heart slips a bit. She flattens her palm against my cheek and gazes at me. "Oh, don't look so glum. It's nothing to be sad over. He asked me out and I said yes. It's hard to pass up a free meal and having something to do. Besides, we aren't exclusive are we?"

"No. I suppose we aren't."

"At least I didn't think we were. So, what about the next night? Then I'll be all yours, darling." She gives me a smile and a grin that brightens me up a bit.

And as our lips press together again and again, I realize that there is no way to pry the lock to her young heart, that it is her beauty to which I fasten myself; it is a cataract upon my reason and makes a lustful creature of me.

Charlotte gone, I close the door to rejoin the party, which is now nearly passed out and gasping for life.

"Let's go for a swim," I yell out, and the party revives itself as we fill William's Honda with six people, and I drive us out to Mercer's Pier.

When we arrive, we run toward the sea, Sean tripping and falling spread eagle in the sand. We shed our shoes, and the beach cools my feet as the water shines black in the moon night. I kick sand with my bare feet and shout as I dive into the water. I tuck my body and plunge into a wave, and then the world is suddenly thick with quiet. When I surface, William paddles over on his back, sprays water from his mouth like a whale, and it showers us.

"That the new girl that came by tonight?" he asks.

"Yeah."

"Well, sounds like things are going well, so why are you keeping her such a secret? You never introduced us."

"No reason."

He spits water again, laughs, then speeds away.

I dip back into the black sea and pretend I'm like the fishes. I listen to the gentle sound of the ocean's sway, the water sloshing me suspended in this strange world. Underwater, my unanchored body floats in quiet blackness. I feel no weight here. I feel nothing but the tug of the current and the swish of my hair. Nearby, muffled laughter reverberates and warbles through the black water I hover in. I listen to the sounds of this other world, the night sea. I am restful. I am happy. I am at peace.

My held breath unable to sustain me any longer, I surface to let my strained lungs breathe again. I gulp in the night air, wipe salt from my eyes, and stare up to a star sky.

Charlotte and I lie on her couch, lazing the afternoon away. I pass her another mint julep. Having bought fresh mint at the downtown market, we have been drinking these for most of the afternoon. Her mother is away and won't be back until tomorrow.

"Be wise and taste," I say as I give her the drink.

We kiss. The tang of alcohol on our lips is like sweet sugar spun from a mouth of mint and cotton candy. We kiss again as a sad, slow song plays in the background.

"Tell me something," she says suddenly. "Tell me something smart from one of those books you've read."

"Well," I say. "What about something from Milton. What if I told you that we shouldn't let time slip away like a neglected rose. That we shouldn't let it wither on the stalk."

She smiles. I slip my hand along her soft arms, follow around her shoulder and slide a tentative grip to her breast. She removes her shirt, her bra, and leans into the chaise lounge and lets out a pleasured sigh of air that is as intoxicating as our juleps. When we move to her room, we slowly unpeel our clothes in the glow of late afternoon.

"Are you sure?" I say breathlessly. "It does seem a little quick."

"Yes," Charlotte says. "I want this."

She passes me a condom and in the humid Wilmington night, we are safe, are quiet, and are together as man and woman were made. Eventually, our passion cooled, our rasping breath tired out, we lie beside one another, returned to the whir of her ceiling fan and the rustling of a warm wind in the trees outside her open window. We are limp with passion, and for a moment happiness seems unassailable, but Charlotte suddenly calls out in pain.

"Are you okay?" I ask, leveling a concerned hand on her back. She draws her knees to her breasts and breathes heavy into her pillow.

"It's some kind of stomach pain," she says. "I suppose I'm just tense," she adds through clenched jaw, stilted breath. She gets up to go to her bathroom and is gone for a short time before returning, still clutching her ailing stomach. "This is bad," she says, breathing timidly.

When she lies back down beside me, I stroke her hair as I would a cat and stare far off to her ceiling tiles, and I wonder what I've done. A tense stillness hovers in the stagnant air between us.

I stay through twilight and into the late hours when night shrouds around us and morning grows closer. We are mostly quiet and do not say much as we eat and then later listen to music. She plays the piano for me, but it is not the same. When she folds down the piano keys' cover, she comes to me, kisses me, and turns her head down to hide her sorrow.

"I'm sorry," she says. "I can't do this."

She puts a soft and beautiful hand to my face. Apologizes until, tears streaming from her eyes, she disappears into the safety of her bedroom.

Her door closes and I sit there for a while, finishing my drink, and then I let myself out and drive home through night's ashen haze while the world around dozes in sleep. I make a desultory loop of the downtown before finally curving around the Oak Cemetery, where a thin mist envelops the marble slabs marking ancient graves. My hope seems interred there, too.

When I arrive home, I shower, and decide sleep is not for me this night, so I drive out again. I pass the estuary that smokes in the coming morning, and I arrive at the ocean pier just as the sky begins to lighten. I lie against the sand, face east, and wait for the day to happen. Soon, the sun peeks over the oceanline and tinges everything blood orange. And then heavy sadness comes. I curl my body on the sand, and, head between my knees as an unborn child, I goddamn it all. I cry out and hurl handfuls of sand into an ocean wind that flicks the grains back into my face. I spread myself out along the beach and sleep as the dawn wind gusts wildly and as the savage sun rises and burns the night away.

CHASE MANHATTAN OWNS ME

OCTOBER 1995. A COOL DAY, SLOW DRIZZLE OUTSIDE. AS I SIT GOING over my bills, I realize my summer expenses have sacked me. With each passing month, my debt spirals further in the red to the point that now I am virtually insolvent. I charge everything: gas; food; toiletries; household supplies; and, necessarily, my medical bills not covered by insurance. When the bills come in the mail, I line them up in order of their due dates, and when the date nears and my bank account is underfunded, I withdraw cash on my credit card to cover the shortage. And then when the charge card requests their payment, I forward the minimum amount.

For several months I have done this, and for several months I get on the American way; I live in debt. But now Chase Manhattan wants to talk to me. They call daily. They leave messages. I am late on my payment, they say. I am over my limit, they add. And now, they are putting a hold on my account.

In college, a Chase Manhattan employee encouraged me to apply for a card (and receive a free pizza!), and as he slipped the sheet of paper for me to sign, he ran a clean hand through his mat of thick black hair. "Now you won't be tied to Mom and Dad's purse strings," he said. "And you can start to work on your credit history, something that will be very important after college when you go to buy a car, a house." In two weeks, the card came. I went into town and bought a guitar, an amp, a distortion pedal, some cords, and threw in a few picks just for good measure. This was happiness. And when I got my college work study paychecks, I signed it over to Chase, and I felt then that I understood economics and how the world of money worked. Now, however, I am shackled to debt, to Chase Manhattan.

"William," I say one night after an evening of endless calculations, "I can't afford living here anymore. I've been going over the bills and the money I owe and I just don't know what to do anymore. I'm broke. I can hardly afford these grilled cheese sandwiches I've been living on. I think it's time I moved."

William nods his head knowingly. "It's been a good ride," he says. "But I'm broke, too. It's coming to an end." He flips a cigarette from his pack and lights it as he leans back into the sofa. I shift the ice pack on my ankle and stare at the silent television, it reflecting the unpaid cable bill.

"I'm just tired," I offer as way of further explanation.

"Well, you look tired, and a little thin, too." He puffs again. "So what are you going to do?"

"I'm not sure. But I'm thinking of resigning from the high school at Christmastime and moving home for a while. I need a way out of this. I have too much debt and my ankles also need a break."

"That's too bad. Nobody really wants to move home. But perhaps it's for the best." He stretches his legs along the couch. "Oh, but it's been a good summer here."

"It has."

William and I have another time out on the town, but it's not the same. We run underneath the clouded moon as the night sky ladles an early winter rain upon us. It freezes my hair as we hurry from Lula's to a late-night dance club. Inside and drying out, I sip a beer and watch the crowd and soon become fascinated with a girl who whips her long blonde hair around and twirls her slender body upon the strobe-lit floor. She is beautiful and I pause to wonder where in the tiny town of New London I'm going to chance upon a girl like this, in a club like this. The girl dances on. The thump of the bass is the beat of my pining heart.

As the last leaves are torn loose by the winter gusts, leaving the trees a husk of naked bark, I pack my belongings and head home. The whole trip it pours rain. White-sharp lightning peals across the dark sky as I drive through Lumberton, Wadesboro, Albemarle, and then into New London.

Mom launches out the front door with an umbrella and rushes me. She scans my truck bed and the blue tarp that bulges with my things. "What's all this?" she asks.

"I'm coming home."

"You are?" She hugs me in a strict and loving squeeze. "I know you don't want to move here," she says. "But I think it is for the best. If you're in as much debt as you say you are, you can save money. Plus your ankles really need time to heal and they can't do that if you keep running yourself into the ground. I think it's a smart move," she says, beginning to grab things from my truck bed. "Besides, I'm sure it's only temporary. It'll give me a little time to fatten you up. You're looking pretty thin these days."

I hoist a suitcase of clothes and carry this inside, tossing it on the floor, and, with Mom's help, I return again and again with armloads of my possessions until, the last box unloaded, I collapse onto my bed. Yet I am not done. Today I must take my monthly dose of Pentamidine. Luckily it is a thing I can now do at home.

I unbox the nebulizer and plug it in and prop it at my bedside. Then I go through the steps of preparing the Pentamidine, which, like my factor, is stored in separate vials of dry powder and saline. I mix the two, draw the medicine into a tiny syringe, dispense it in the aerosol canister, and bring the mouthpiece to my lips. I breathe in the drug, breathe out. And when the medicine is spent—the mouthpiece no longer puffing white smoke—I realize that I need to factor. My ankle throbs and gives when I stand. The move has worn my body down.

I prepare my factor, wait, treat, and then curl onto my bed, holding my breath for the pain. I slip underneath the covers, let air into the sheets, and comfort my ankle atop a pillow, and then I don't move. I try to make myself as still as the night and to sleep as best I can. Yet I stare around my moonlit room at the outdated posters and high school memorabilia pinned to the walls, and suddenly a morose lump clogs my throat. I feel I have not moved on, but have returned again to senior year. I have gone out in the world and tried to make something of myself, and I have failed and have now returned.

I brace my ankle against the ice pack, shift, and sleep while the specters of the past hold court at my bedside.

Christmas Day, just as the winter sun fades from the cold sky, Dad lights a fire in our den, and I pull a rocking chair next to it and warm my feet on the hearth while I begin a new book. Dad sits beside me and watches the fire flame while upstairs I can hear Mom, Anne, and Louise trying on their new Christmas outfits and making gasps and exclamations of excitement.

"Now, Son," Dad says to me. I mark my book with my thumb and look over to him. "I know you're down in the mouth about having to come home and all, but I just thought you should know that your mother," he says, taking a sip of his Maker's Mark, "your mother is tickled pink about your being home. She's been like a kid this Christmas, about to wet her pants she's so happy . . . It's been lonely here for her, I know, with me having to work in Goldsboro during the week, you off to school, and with Anne doing her thing up there at NC State. This house gets mighty quiet during the week with just your mom and Louise here. I know that. Hell, I think if she thought it would keep you here longer, she woulda bought the whole goddamn bookstore for you at Christmas." He sips again. Ice clinks in his glass. "Now listen to me, Son," he says. "I want you to do something for me. You think you can do that?"

I nod that I can.

Dad stands up and stokes the fire with the poker. Flames rise and a sudden whistle of gas pops from one of the logs and plumes out a blue-yellow dance of fire. "Goddamn it," he yells suddenly as ash spews out onto the hearth. He jumps quickly, spills some of his drink. I jerk away my feet from the sparks.

"You okay?" he asks.

"Yeah. I'm fine. It's nothing. Just startled me." He rests the poker against the fireplace, settles back into his chair with his drink. "Now, Son. What I want you to do is to take one, two, maybe three days—hell, you might need a whole week—but what I want you to do, Son, is to think about what you really wanna do. What is it you wanna do with your life? Now, I know you've been doing this teaching and that you've had your insurance and had a pretty good time living your life down there in Wilmington, but you know and I know that you can't be doing that your whole life, now can you?"

"I don't know. I guess not. I haven't thought about it."

"That's my point." Dad's eyes grow large and aware. "Son, it's time. Think about it. You can't work like other people. You're different. You need to find something that fits for you and all you're up against. Your mom and I can't be here forever for you to come home to, you know."

I lean forward in my chair and I open my mouth to speak, but Dad quiets me.

"Tsst, tsst, tsst," he says, stilling me with his upraised hand. "I don't want you to answer me. Not today. I just wanted you to think about it. Can you do that? Your mom and I know that you're too smart to keep killing yourself as a teacher's assistant. That's no life for you. Just think about it, okay. Promise me that."

"Okay. I promise."

"All right, then." He swishes his ice, swallows diluted whiskey. "Now, I've gotta go and re-freshen this," he says pointing to his glass. "Watch that fire for me while I'm gone."

When he ascends the stairs, I return to my book. The fire crackles and warms the den and it burns heat until well past midnight when it eventually extinguishes into a warm orange glow. I hear the natural creak of a floorboard, but then nothing but palpable quiet. I close my book and in my new journal, I write:

> *Christmas 1995. Rain, no snow, but very cold. 12:45 in the a.m.*
> *I love that—"in the a.m." Sounds like something Henry James might*
> *write. Has a nice ring to it. The house sleeps, the fire nearby dies out,*
> *I write. I am home.*
>
> *Received several gifts today: books, clothes, strings for my guitar,*
> *a pocket watch, and this leather journal which has the inscription,*
> *"Thought you might have some time to write. Love, Mom and Dad."*

So I write tonight. Record, I suppose, the events of today.

In the morning the family opened presents. Anne loved the sweater I got her, Louise the Hulk video. Dad seemed mildly amused by his Nicorette gum, but asserted that he'd yet be ever faithful to his Marlboros, a habit which, I fear, shall buy his coffin for sure. I gave Mom some fancy coffee which she quickly brewed and we both savored.

Later, my aunts, uncles, and cousins arrived and we ate a late meal and dozed off the afternoon before they all left. Then Dad entertained me with a speech which encouraged me to consider my future. I guess all sons must get that kind of advice from their breadwinning fathers. It was the low point of the day.

Read a story by Chekhov, another by Cheever—it seems my parents must have shopped heavily in the bookstore's "C" aisle—but was then consumed by Braudel's History of the Mediterranean *also given to me for Christmas. Braudel's prose is good, clean, and vivid. His description of the Mediterranean Sea and the snow-capped Alps rising along the horizon momentarily transported me. Oh . . . to be there. Instead of here for as long as I fear I might be. I give it five months. Maybe six. At least until summer, I suppose. It all depends on how long it will take my part-time job—which I haven't gotten yet—to pay down my debt. My debt—that's another thing I should write down here sometime. How it happened. How it came to be so enormous. Perhaps I'll save that for another winter day. As for Braudel's history, I'm not far into yet, but am already enthralled and think it grand. It is a good day when you find something like that.*

So, I suppose ole Mom and Dad were right—that I would have time to write in this journal. What else is there to do but write and think in a sleepy little town like this? But there is comfort and solace in this, in writing. It makes me feel better somehow. Perhaps I should stop then before I uncover something of a sadder, darker nature. Hmmm . . . Okay . . . Good-night.

ANKLES

February 1996. In the hospital X-ray room, the lanky technician asks me to turn my left ankle out for his photo. Tall and angular, his skin is blanched and in want of sunlight, and although his manner is courteous and professional, he is brisk and offers very little in the way of conversation as he twists me into position. He says nothing of my ankle's size, but grabs and positions it at an unnatural angle.

"Okay. That's good. Hold it. Hold it."

He hurries off—a stick with fast legs—behind his protective shield and presses his button. Then he repeats the process for my other, less swollen ankle, but this time when he jerks me, I wince.

"I'm sorry, but the orthopedist asked that I get a good shot of your joint. It's a difficult angle." So, I endure. Grit my teeth and let out a slow rasp of air.

Once handed my X-ray charts, I return to the orthopedic clinic where I wait next to an elderly man, his leg plastered in a milky cast. We smile at one another, but say nothing, and he is soon called and crutches away in slow arthritic unhaste. Eventually I am taken back, and when the orthopedist shows, he shakes my hand. This orthopedist is new and young and tall and blessed with a thick turf of brown hair that is short and combed back in a wave. Additionally, he is talkative so that in the few minutes it takes for him to enter the room, thumb through my folder, glance at my recent X-rays, scrub his hands, and then adjust his tie by securing it inside his shirt pocket—he relates his youthful career as a fledgling football tackle.

"I wasn't any kind of star," he offers with a humbling smile, "but it all led to what I was supposed to do. This." He spreads open his arms in a gesture meant to encompass the room and designate it as his chosen profession, and it is then that I note his stocky build, something like a square with thick legs and arms.

He approaches, scrutinizes my ankle with a searching glance, and when he asks me to walk, I lower myself from the table and, shoeless, pad up and down the carpeted hallway as he studies my hobbled gait. We return to the room, and as he proceeds to further examine me, I catch the sporty lingo peppered in his dialogue, no doubt a result of his deep affinity for athletics. Stooping over to better see my ankle and rolling it around in his hand, the orthopedist jokingly tells me that it is like a warped football.

"You can play with it, but it's not ideal. That ankle is choked with fluid. We're going to need a game plan for it because if we don't come up with something your touchdown days are going to be over. You're walking by flexing what we call your lumbricals." In explaining this, he adopts a more sophisticated, medical tone. "Lumbricals are the small muscles in your feet. You've got them in your hands, too, but at any rate, you're not using those in your ankle. You're bending more with your foot bones." He turns my joint in my hands, causing me to jump from the pain. "Sorry about that."

He rises and, pointing to the light-box where my X-rays are displayed, illuminates my ankle's degeneration, the arthritis that has set in, and the bone spur that has developed, a condition that contributes to the sharp and shooting pain I've complained about. He goes on a bit more and then concludes with his game: surgery. "An operation would fuse the joint," he says, "and would slow down your joint's bleeding since it will remove the tissue from between it. Consequently, your swelling should be less and so should the pain."

"Will I be able to walk?"

"Of course, you'll be able to walk. It'll take some time, and with a fused ankle you won't ever be what I'd call 'normal' because, well, your ankle will no longer bend, but you certainly could easily hold for the placekicker. I have no doubts about that."

"Well, how long am I looking at being in the hospital?" I'm thinking about the operation on my right knee in 1980 and the eight weeks it took to recover and the other done in 1982 and the seven-week hospital stay required.

"Shouldn't be too long. No more than a week. Like the time between one double-header Saturday and the next."

"A week? Wow. I'm used to these things taking several weeks."

"Yeah. Medicine's come a long way."

I agree on the surgery, and in late spring, I return for my presurgery evaluation. The orthopedist enters with printouts of my lab work. The blood drawn, the tests run, and my health translated into numbers, the orthopedist surveys the results that are unfolded in his lap like an unbound book. He rolls his chair next to me, grabs my ankle in his hand, feels around again, then backs away to reconsult my chart. He rubs his chin.

"I'm not sure you're ready for surgery. We may have to take a rain date on this one. It's a tough call." He folds his hands in his lap. "We got your tests back, and your counts have dropped below a safe level for operating." He looks up. "I always knew your HIV was a factor, but in a person with these counts, I think that the risk for infection is just too high. I think I'm going to bench you." He breathes heavy. Pushes away. "If things improve," he goes on, "we'll run an audible, but for now it's best to sit you on the sidelines and keep an eye on things."

I squeeze my hands together. I lower my head, stare down at my softball ankle. "What am I supposed to do?"

"We'll treat the pain and see how that goes. But don't get too down about this little setback. On the bright side, I've been studying your X-rays and there's a good possibility your ankles may fuse themselves. They definitely are closing that gap and drawing the bones together. I've seen it happen. Sometimes, if you leave it alone, the body takes care of itself."

He stands, writes out a prescription for Vicodin, and then pumps my hand up and down in a vigorous shake. "It's just not your day to be on the field."

At home after I deliver the news, Mom quiets. "Well . . . I guess it just wasn't meant to be," she says.

She embraces me in a warm hug, and then we go inside and pour ourselves cups of coffee and sit at the kitchen table. We say little to one another but instead watch through the window as the spring sun descends into our backyard and beyond into the vacant barnlot and barren pasture. Mom spins her mug in her hands. Her wedding ring clinks against the porcelain handle as she drums her nervous fingers against the cup.

THE DEPRESSING EFFECT

OF NUMBERS

July 1996. Hot. Very hot. The sun—a hazy orb of melting heat—parboils the trees and flowers. They weep. But I rest in the cool hospital room, tired and dozing while waiting for Dr. Trum. When he enters, he startles me. I brush my shirt and shorts flat, raise my arms in an exaggerated yawn, and position myself for the examination. Dr. Trum cleans his hands and asks me to remove my socks so that he can see my ankles, and like the orthopedist, he cups the rotund left one and passes a probing thumb across its swelling. He inquires about the pain medicine and, though I hurt and limp daily, I allow that the narcotic has aided some. My pain when I walk is now endurable.

"I was sorry to hear about that operation," he offers. "But I agree with the orthopedist. It's not a risk worth taking. Your CD4 counts have dropped below fifty."

"What's normal?"

"Oh, it's hard to say. It fluctuates. But perhaps a thousand is a likely number."

He feels my lymph nodes by kneading his hands underneath my arms and along my neck as if I were bread, and he tells me that they're inflamed and that this is a sign of my declining immunity. There is nothing to do about it, he adds. It is only a sign.

He shines a light in my eyes and asks about my visit to the ophthalmologist: "Any floaters?" he asks.

"None so far," I answer.

"That's good. Very good."

And in my mouth, he rolls the tongue depressor around and then traps my tongue with it while he examines my throat with his tiny flashlight.

"Thrush," he pronounces. "You have thrush. We don't want that spreading down your throat and causing problems with eating. You don't need that." My face droops. My eyes feel blue and watery. "It's nothing to worry over yet. It's just a sign of your declining immunity. We'll give you a rinse for that. No sweat."

He turns to my folder and asks me if I'm keeping up with my Pentamidine; I answer that I am. "Now that you're doing it at home, it's up to you to remember it."

"I'm keeping up. No missed doses."

"Good. Very good," he says again. "Don't need you catching pneumonia."

Then he leans back and then forward and, staring me down, explains that he is recommending me to the Infectious Disease Clinic. "With them on board and with us working on this together to prevent infections, I feel our chances are better. After all, I'm just a hematologist who became involved with HIV when all this was breaking and coming down the pipeline. You might say, I'm sort of a backdoor study. That doesn't mean I'm not capable. I just think that more heads are better than one. And the ID Clinic are the up-and-coming experts here." He shuffles my file. "I would suggest restarting you on AZT and see how that might improve things, but I know your aversion for it and, happily, I'm hopeful about what I've been reading in the current literature about a new way to treat HIV with protease inhibitors. I think if we can get you to hold on—that is getting plenty of rest, eating well, exercising, and keeping a close eye on you to stop any infections before they become problematic—I think if we can do this, then, once the FDA approves the inhibitors, you may have a good shot here at beating this thing. The inhibitors aren't an end-all cure, but I think it's something to work towards."

Immediately, my mood grows dark and afraid. It has been almost six years since I was told of my HIV, at least fourteen if not more since I was infected through my transfusions, and now it comes to this. HIV has sacked my immunity and left me with only a shaky defense like some flimsy buckler gripped before my heart.

I let myself off the table and go to the ID Clinic, where I again fall asleep while waiting. I cannot say how much time passes with my head leaned back at a crooked angle and my light snore filling the waiting room, but eventually I feel upon my shoulder the gentle touch of a nurse who holds my chart. She is slender and pretty, and I force a weak smile for her.

"The doctor'll see you now," she says.

I am led through the hallway and then weighed, temperatured, and blood pressured and am then deposited in another room to wait. Still tired, I sleep again, but it is not long before the doctor wakes and examines me. In silence, he roams his hands across my swollen lymph nodes and studies the thrush in my mouth.

"Your CD4 counts are quite low," he says. "Are you experiencing any problems like fever, night sweats, difficulty breathing?"

"Only that thrush. But other than that, no. Not really any problems. I'm just tired. Really, really tired."

"Hmmm. Well, that could be something starting in you."

"What?"

"Well, I'm not sure. It may be nothing. But I think you should plan on coming here once a month to get blood work and see me. I need to follow you closely." He pauses, reaches to a desk folder, and passes me a packet. "Also, I'm worried about your weight. What's normal for you?"

"Oh, I don't know. One forty-five or so, I guess."

"Well, you're down to 128. We need to bring that back up. Inside that packet I just gave you, there's a sheet outlining diet supplements that will help. Yogurt shakes and picking up cans of Ensure can really add weight to you and help fight off infections. You should read through it. It should give you advice on things to eat and things not to eat like raw fish. Also, I think I'd avoid traveling if you can. Do you travel for work? Or are you planning on vacationing anywhere before summer ends, especially somewhere like Mexico where the sanitation is pretty poor?"

"No. No plans."

"Okay, then. So that's not a problem."

"No, I suppose not."

"Then I'll see you back in a month."

In this way, our visit ends. From the pharmacy, I pick up the medicinal rinse for thrush and a case of the recommended Ensure.

As the days and weeks pass, a depressive cloud overtakes me and I become a dispirited vessel of routine. On the days I don't work the few hours of respite care for an autistic boy, I wake at eight and lie in bed until nine, ten, and sometimes eleven. I throw out the coffee Mom leaves for me in the pot—it is usually scorched from sitting out so long—and I brew more and, from the dining room, I watch as the sun evaporates the dew from the night before and bronzes the once-green grass. At this point, if there is any morning left, I read until it feels late, and then I travel into town for lunch and then to the library, where I read the papers and write in my journal. For weeks, Monday becomes Tuesday, Thursday, and then another Monday. My heart pumps. Blood flows in, cycles out. I breathe.

LOOSE LIPS

August 1996. When I move to Chapel Hill, I am more alone, more depressed than I have ever been. It is as if a melancholic miasma trails me and makes a blue cloud upon my heart. If for no other reason than to leave my parents' and to shake off the idea I have of myself as a failure—a thing reinforced by my living at home—I have moved here. A friend who went to college at UNC said it was a nice place to live. Another concurred. And after visiting, I decided it as good a place as any to move. Yet Mom is against it. Before I drove away, she pleaded for me to stay: "You need to take care of yourself," she said. "Why can't you stay a little longer?"

"I just can't." And I pulled away.

I accept an assistant's position at Aster Elementary and in August settle into a tiny apartment, two miles from the school. Here there is only me and the blue carpet that covers the floors. Outside, stout evergreens fence my home and their dark boughs block out light. The cell of pine and the blue, blue carpet—throughout, the color is blue—make me sad for no other reason than I am encoffined by this shade.

I soon discover that I am cut off from my neighbors by language. They speak Spanish; I do not. So we nod at one another when we pass or when we lock our doors tight beside the other, and at night I calculate their footfalls on the floor above me, reckoning that they are eight or nine or perhaps as many as ten living in a similarly small blue apartment as me. They rise early, work late, stay to themselves, and are from a country I long to visit. They are the only company I know.

At Aster Elementary, I am assigned to Thomas, an autistic first grader. He is part of the public schools' move toward inclusion: integrating handicapped students in "normal" classroom environments instead of isolating them from the student body, as is the typical case. Endlessly irascible, Thomas likes to punch students, throw crayons, and kick whatever might be in his feet's path.

On my first morning, Thomas slumps at his desk while Mrs. Price—the first-grade teacher whose classroom Thomas and I are placed in—goes over vocabulary words. Already, I am fatigued. I spent yesterday afternoon at another ID Clinic visit, bought a few groceries, and then went home to take my monthly Pentamidine dose before dinner and then bedtime. I yawn. I encourage Thomas:

"Please do your work, Thomas. You won't get recess. Please do your work."

Thomas tries to stab me with his pencil and then tosses it across the room, interrupting the lesson. Mrs. Price stops to admonish Thomas and me.

"Thomas, stop," she reproaches. "Mr. Smoak, you need to keep him under control. He is *your* responsibility," she says to me. In a meeting we had the day before—one of several—Mrs. Price acknowledged she only allowed Thomas in her classroom because of a promise that, with an assistant, he would be handled. In this way, she constantly reminds me of my job. "Perhaps you should take Thomas outside and let him calm down."

"Yes, ma'am."

I yawn again when we are outside.

At noontime, I lunch with Thomas. I insert the straw into his juice box, unwrap the bologna sandwich his mother packed, and open his bag of chips—all while keeping a close eye on him, as he loves throwing food. At the undersized table made for children, I squeeze into the plastic seat and nibble my own lunch while around me, children talk loudly with their mouths open; the cinder-block room rumbles with a chittery-chattery roar that would give anyone borderline tinnitus. Soon a lady walks over and extends her hand as she joins us.

"Catherine. Catherine Eaves. I'm a second-grade teacher here. And those," she says pointing at a nearby table, "are my little young'uns." She begins to unbag her lunch. In her mid-fifties, she has blonde-white hair done up on top and wears thick glasses rimmed in brown. Her long gold earrings dangle loosely above her shoulders, and she wears a black shirt with a lively embroidered pattern raised on it. "So, is this your first day, honey?"

"Yes."

"Going okay for you?"

"So-so, I suppose. I'm getting by and learning the ropes."

"Well, I hope you still don't think this is an elementary school because it's not. Really it's more like a country club. At least that's what some of the teachers think."

"Oh, really. I hadn't caught on to that yet."

"Well, you will. And you have to be asked to join their club. Have you been asked yet?" she teases while taking a bite of her carrot.

"Well, no. At least I don't believe so."

"I doubt it. Or you'd be sitting with them at their table instead of here all alone with Thomas."

"Well, I have to keep an eye on him." We both look over to Thomas who chews and stares off at the ceiling. "But then, why aren't you with them?"

"Oh, honey. They hate me. Absolutely can't stand me." She leans in closer and lowers her voice so as to not be overheard. "But I know they're just jealous since I'm the only one with my head screwed on straight." Her eyes widen and a little laugh whistles from her tightened red lips, and immediately I trust her.

When we finish our meals and I rise to leave, Catherine lightly grabs my arm. "Listen to me, honey. A word to the wise. Watch your back. Some here are nothing more than glorified high-schoolers. They're still imagining that they're captain of the cheerleading squad, and they don't care two hoots about anybody else. Just watch yourself. Keep your head low and do what you're told and you'll be fine."

In September, I am swimming in the depths of fatigue. I dream of dreaming, of having that luxury. Yesterday, I returned to the ID Clinic and the week before I saw both the ophthalmologist and Dr. Trum, and I was tired then as my ankles thumped with pain and my mouth yawned for rest. I napped in the waiting rooms and then upon the examination tables. Assigned to bus duty, I now rub my eyes and I watch the children unload from the buses and spill into the cafeteria for breakfast. An unseasonably cool wind blows. I cough. Snot runs from my nose as I cough again, blow.

After lunch, I deposit Thomas at speech therapy and walk to my supervisor's office adjacent to the school's playground. It is time for my first review. Although I'm a bit nervous, I've been through such things before at New Hanover High School, and it always went well. At the meeting, my supervisor is informal and jovial. We vent about Thomas's behavior and laugh a bit while we firm up his classroom goals. My supervisor concludes our meeting by suggesting that I communicate more frequently with Thomas's mother. "Send notes home," she offers, "or chat a bit more in the parking lot when she picks Thomas up after school." She sips her diet soda. "His mother calls here every other day," she says with raised eyebrows and a deep sigh expressing her annoyance. "What can you do, right?" She sips again. "Otherwise, I feel you're doing a terrific job with Thomas. I know he can be hard to work with and it takes a lot of patience, but you're getting him controlled. We're glad to have you here. Not everybody can do this job; that's for sure."

I leave her office feeling that something in my life may be going right.

In the afternoon before school officially lets out, I meet Thomas's mom in the parking lot and update her on his day. She seems pleased and talks right up until the bell rings and I must excuse myself for afternoon bus duty. I hurry to the pickup zone and gather the waiting children against the benches and watch as young mothers arrive and tug their loved ones away. When a fight breaks out between two fifth-graders, I wedge my thin body between them and pull down their tender fists before they can inflict bruises, and then I isolate them. When they settle, I hear a woman's voice behind me.

"Excuse me, don't I know you?" I turn around to a mother who stands with two boys swinging from her arms. "Are you Shelby? Shelby Smoak?"

"Yes, I am."

The lady extends her hand. "Cindy. Cindy Reed. I used to work in the

Hemophilia Center at the hospital. Don't you remember me? You were just a little boy then, probably about ten or eleven."

I have a vague memory of her. "Oh, yes. It's been a long time. How are you?"

"Fine, fine. Just picking up my two boys." She lifts their hands in pride. "Do you work here?"

"Yes. An assistant in first grade."

"Oh." She stiffens. "How wonderful." Pause. "And how's your mom?"

"Fine."

"Your dad, too?"

"Fine."

"Sister, was it Anne?"

"And Louise and they're both fine."

"Well that's good to hear." She starts toward her car and turns around one last time, giving me a strange backwards glance. "You take care of yourself, okay."

"I will." And I can feel it—her knowing about me. And I feel something else, too—something unkind about that look she gives me.

But the boys are at it again and distract me from my thoughts. I rush over, force them apart, and escort them into Principal Trask's office, where they are reprimanded and then returned to me with drawn-down faces and notes in their grip. When their rides arrive, I tell Johnny's brother about his behavior, for which his brother gives Johnny a quick slap on the back of the scalp and a stern warning; Billy's mother jerks him by the arm and yanks him to the car, scolding him until the car door slams and shuts out her yelling. Then eventually, only one remains, a second-grader with her hair braided and pulled into one long blonde pigtail.

"Are you sure you have a ride?"

"Yes. Mommy is usually late. This one time, she was almost two hours late."

"Oh great," I say.

Chelsea miffs her face. "That's not great. That's bad."

"Yes, I know. I was being funny."

"Oh." She looks at me with befuddled eyes.

When we have waited forty minutes, I suggest that we go inside; it's growing cold and I need to use the phone in Principal Trask's office. There, I call all Chelsea's numbers—home, mother's work, father's work, and then emergency—but only the machines are answering. I leave messages. Then I sit and wait. Chelsea reads a book while I flip through a school newsletter. Soon the teachers begin filing out, leaving. "Oh, bus duty," one says as she passes. "There's always one parent that just ruins it. Gotta love it."

The assistant principal soon emerges and checks his watch with the hall clock. "Yep, they're late." He smiles. "Who knows? You may still be here tomorrow."

After another half hour, I bother Principal Trask and again phone Chelsea's numbers.

"No luck?" Principal Trask asks.

"Nope. No luck."

I return to the hallway with Chelsea and wait again.

More time passes before Principal Trask comes out to see how things are. He stands over me and, as way of conversation, tells me the good things he's heard about me from my supervisor. While he talks, he smoothes down his red tie and works his arms into a light gray suit-jacket, which he adjusts for a better fit. But I can't take my eyes off of his crooked nose. Once broken, it now gives him a sinister look, no matter how often he smiles.

"Somebody'll be here soon for her," he encourages. "Can't be much longer now." He smoothes back his hair. "Wanna make a few more calls before I lock up?" he asks.

"No. I've left enough messages."

"Okay then."

He turns the key to the office and then he is gone. Later, the janitor sweeps around us while Chelsea sleeps on a wooden bench pressed against the trophy wall, scrunching up her bookbag for a pillow.

Eventually, daylight fading from the sky, a car pulls through the drive; a woman rushes in, darts her eyes around, and quickly lets out a sigh when she spots Chelsea sleeping upon the bench.

"Oh, thank God. I was sure you would have sent her home in a taxi by now. I got caught at work and just couldn't get away." She advances. "Chelsea . . . Chelsea," she calls.

Chelsea screws up her eyes, "Mommy?"

Her mother kneels down and rubs a hand along Chelsea's back. "Oh, honey. I'm so sorry. Mommy got caught at work. I couldn't help it, but I'm here now. Let's go home, okay? Let's go home and I'll fix your favorite dinner."

Chelsea polishes sleep from her eyes and collects her things.

"I hope Chelsea wasn't any trouble for you," the mother says, offering a smile.

I grit my anger. "If you're late like this again, she'll have to start riding the bus."

Chelsea's mother vilifies me with her eyes. "It happens," she says.

Then she carts Chelsea away in a half-sleep, and I go home to rest, falling straight into bed and skipping supper, only to be awakened by the phone later: my mom. Playing the good son, I chat, venting about the horrors of bus duty and then mentioning my encounter with my former nurse.

"You ran into Cindy Reed?" Mom inquires.

"Yeah. She's got kids at Aster."

"Oh, Lord . . ." Mom swallows. "You know she was let go from the Hemophilia Center for talking too much."

"Talking. About what?"

"Well, that's when everything was just coming out, and, well, Cindy couldn't keep things to herself. She couldn't keep quiet is all I heard. She was young and a little immature for the situation and, well, she just liked to talk. At least that's what I heard."

"Well, I'm sure things have changed."

"I hope so, Son. For your sake. I hope so. You just watch out. That's her kids at that school."

One Friday in the middle of October, my supervisor blocks me in the hallway and, nearly out of breath, tells me that she has been looking for me and that we're scheduled for a meeting today.

"Oh. Okay. I didn't know."

"You wouldn't have. This is an impromptu meeting. Can you meet me in thirty minutes?" she asks brusquely.

"Yes. Sure."

And thirty minutes later when I enter my supervisor's office, she rushes for the door with her arms strapped around a stack of paperwork.

"Are we going somewhere?"

"We're actually meeting in the principal's office today. He's got some available time, and he likes to sit in on these things when he can. Also, it's good for him to be part of the review."

We are quiet as we walk the corridor of napping kindergarten children. My supervisor's pants' fabric swishes and her heels click as we make haste to the principal's office. My gut stirs.

Reclined behind his desk and talking on the phone, Principal Trask motions for us to come in and sit at a small table near his desk. I listen as he laughs and ends the conversation, and when he hangs up, he immediately goes to close the door.

"Glad you could meet on such short notice." He extends his hand and offers me a polite shake before adjusting his tie and settling next to my supervisor and across from me. "We get so busy around here, we have to squeeze things in when we can." He opens a folder that I catch my name on, and he asks me to tell him how I feel things with Thomas are going.

"Okay. Thomas has definitely calmed down since the first of the year."

"That's good to hear." Principal Trask leans forward, points to a sheet of paper my supervisor holds. "I'm meeting with you today because we haven't really had time to thoroughly go over your objectives and duties for the position you've been hired for. We've just now printed out a copy of your job requirements and felt this was as good a time as any to update you on your progress. This is our way of keeping things on track and letting you know where you stand." He gives my supervisor a go-ahead glance and she begins.

"As you know Thomas is a special case. A special boy needing extra-special care." She lays the paper flat, toys with her fingers. Her voice is like a tiny stream of air slipping from a balloon, weak and barely audible. "One of the first things he looks for is the attitude of others, especially his assistant."

"You're going to have to speak up, Mrs. Steele. If I can hardly hear you and I'm sitting right next to you, I know Mr. Smoak can't hear you."

"Okay. Okay." She nervously clears her throat and begins again with a more assertive tone. Principal Trask settles back into his seat. "When George, excuse me, I mean Mr. Mitchell . . . when Mr. Mitchell worked with Thomas, they were always rolling around, laughing and cutting up, and generating the kind of connection an autistic boy like Thomas needs. Yet after talking with Mrs. Price, we feel you are not making these same kinds of connections with Thomas."

I'm taken aback. This isn't good.

"Oh." I clear my own throat. I shift my feet beneath the desk and sink into the chair. "I didn't know this was a problem. Last time we talked, you only mentioned improving communication with his mother, and I've tried that."

"Yes, yes," offers Principal Trask. "There has been improvement there. This other is a more recent observation."

I swallow. My supervisor continues.

"Your relationship with Thomas is weak. There doesn't seem to be that respect coming from Thomas to you." Here I think of jumping in to defend myself, but she pipes away, not raising her eyes to notice me. "Number 3," she continues, her voice stern and gaining strength. "You also fail to properly carry Thomas through his daily routine. For example, checking his duty board before allowing him to read a book or making sure that Thomas completes his writing assignment before taking him to bounce on his ball or swing on the playground. Again, we feel that you achieve poorly here."

My supervisor prattles on, enumerating my poor achievements. Her hands tremble. Her voice quavers. And she does not look at me. Principal Trask also averts his eyes and only watches the supervisor reading. I give a hard stare to his crooked nose—it now appearing even more crooked—and I lower my gaze and admire the lace of my shoes, the droop of my tie, the crack in the floor, the drip of my tears on my khakis.

When the supervisor's droning voice ends, Principal Trask speaks: "What we try to achieve here at Aster Elementary is the best teaching environment for our students. One that encourages optimal learning. And after discussing it with Mrs. Steele and Mrs. Price, it seems to me that you may be missing that mark." I sense their eyes probing me. "Typically after making an employee aware of their deficiencies, we reconvene in another week to reevaluate the situation. If at that time we sense no change, then we have to consider a replacement." He leans back in his chair, throws his legs out from under the desk. "You should try to put your best foot forward because we want you to be successful at Aster Elementary and to be a part of our family, don't we, Mrs. Steele?"

She coughs to regain her voice. "Yes, sir. That's right."

"But if you can't meet that mark, then we're going to have to let you go."

My eyes water again. Principal Trask pushes a box of tissue toward me and I take one to clean my face.

"Is there anything you'd like to say?"

"No, sir." I blow my nose.

"Is there anything you'd like to add, Mrs. Steele?"

"No, sir."

He looks to his watch and shakes it around his arm to where he can read its face. "Well, it's two o'clock now. Perhaps it would be best if you took the rest of the day off. I know you're upset and may need to think these things through. Teaching isn't for everyone, especially when you're working with the handicapped." He stands from his chair, moves to the other side of the room. "We'll get someone to look after Thomas this afternoon."

"I have bus duty, too."

"Mrs. Steele, do you think you could cover that this afternoon?"

"Yes, sir. I can do that."

"Great."

And from his desk, Principal Trask draws out a sheet of paper that I am made to sign.

"This just validates our meeting and acknowledges your understanding of what was discussed here."

Then he opens the door and I am let out.

When I slink home to sob, my apartment is bluer than it has ever been. The wind rustles the leaves that cling desperately to their treetops, and through the open window the smell of dying fall drifts in. A hole inside me is now stopped up with a great sorrow.

I fall asleep, and when I wake, the day has darkened. An evening cloud covers the sun. I sit on my bedside, rest my feet on the floor, place my palms flat against my mattress, and I peer outside to the trees and a stormy sky. I turn on the porch light and sit outside while a storm starts to rage around me. Gusts bend the treetops into parabolic arches, tearing loose the last leaves, and when one catches beneath my foot, I pick it up and close my grip around it. Dry, it crumbles in my hand and is blown to nothing in the violent wind.

Sunday evening, I type in the dim light my apartment offers. I rework every line of my resignation letter—a jeremiad of anger, confusion, and, of course, sadness. All weekend, I have thought on this letter. Of what to say. I have wondered how much of my situation is a result of my encounter with Cindy Reed. (This is, necessarily, Mom's firm suspicion.) But then, I am divided between that and the possibility I am really just an unfit teacher's assistant. At New Hanover, I was a good teacher. Nonetheless, this job is spoiled for me; I can no longer work at Aster Elementary.

Early Monday morning, I arrive before the students and deliver my resignation letter to Principal Trask.

"Perhaps this is for the best," he says as he turns it over in his hands. The flap of paper fills up the awkward silence. "There are a ton of professions out there, and teaching isn't for everyone." He avoids my eyes. He shows no hint of regret or sorrow.

I say I will work through Friday. He says that will be fine. I say I am sorry it did not work out. He says he's sorry, too. I request that my letter be put in my file. He says he'll do that. I say good-bye. He says good luck.

And when Friday arrives, there is no party, no farewell. At the day's end, I help Thomas into his parent's van, smile, and politely introduce my replacement who has spent the day with me and Thomas, preparing to take over. I wave good-bye to Thomas and gather my things.

In the parking lot, I take one last look around. I unlock my cab door, but hear my name called and turn to see Catherine Eaves coming toward me in a hasty jog.

"Wait. Wait," she calls out. "I have something for you." She nears and catches her breath. "These are for you," she says, shoving me a Tupperware container. "That's just some brownies I made."

"You shouldn't have done that. Thanks."

"Well, you need to eat. And those are pretty good, if I do say so myself." She lowers her eyes, tightens her brow, and looks at me with concern. "Is it true?"

"Yes, it's true. I've resigned."

"No. I know that. The other. Is it true?"

My heart slows; an icy shudder chills me. "You know?"

"Well, let's just say that the rumors are flying in the country club."

"I see."

She draws her heel in the gravel. A leaf falls between us.

"You don't have to tell me. But I want you to know that I only wish you the best. And although I'll miss our lunches together, you're better off." She pushes a strand of hair from her eye. "I just hate it happened like this. And I hate, too, all the things I hear, especially if they're true." She leans in for a hug. "Just take care of yourself, honey. Please do that. Promise me that, okay?"

"Okay. I promise."

"Okay, honey. I'll miss you, but don't come back here. You hear me. Write this place off."

She gives me a last wave as I accelerate onto Aster Drive toward home. The school disappears until only a tinge of red brick pokes through the woods, and then this contracts and disappears. The fall leaves rustle beneath my tires and the wind sounds lonesome in the bare October trees. And in the night, more rain comes and patters its sad lullaby upon the earth.

THE UNICORN

HALLOWEEN 1996. I ATTEND A PARTY HOSTED BY JAKE, A SOMETIMES friend of mine. Too tired and uncaring to put much thought in my costume, I purchase a mechanic's shirt from the PTA thrift store and, as if I have spent my days rolled underneath cars, I smudge kohl upon my shirt, jeans, and face, decorating myself as a greasy mechanic.

Jake rents an apartment that is hard to find, so by the time I arrive, the party is abuzz with laughter and swaying bodies in costume. I press through the tiny den and scan masks and made-up faces for any that I may know. Eventually, I happen upon Jake, a furry gorilla doing a beer bong through his costume's snout. When he finishes, Jake dances an apish jig and hoots and moans as a gorilla might while people applaud and shout out happy cheers. Noticing me, he pulls me further into the crowd, and, introducing me to his friends along the route, we soon squeeze onto a small balcony where the keg rests. He pumps a cup for me and for himself, and we toast one another, slapping plastic against plastic, and then he abandons me, returns to the party to find his girlfriend dressed up as Jane for the evening. With nothing better to do, I drink more beer as partygoers loop about the keg.

A young girl dressed as a unicorn fills her cup and stands on the balcony, gazing out to the stand of pine edging the back and showing no intention of returning inside. White strings dangle as a mane down her back. She has sewn on a tail and painted a party hat as a spiraled golden horn for her head. Draped in pure white, she appears before me as that creature from those magical books I read so long ago.

"I love unicorns," I say as a way to strike up a conversation.

She looks at me bemusedly, flutters her long unicorn lashes. "Really. Well, this isn't just any unicorn, you know. It's magical."

"That's good because I could use a little magic right now."

"Seems to me that a mechanic could fix just about anything."

"Anything, I suppose, without a heart and lungs."

When she looks to me, her walnut eyes, full of expression, seem brightened by hope. As the night lengthens, we ask questions about the universities we attended, the degrees we hold, and the pastimes we enjoy, and we talk about the people we know in town, hoping to find someone in common, some connection we may have outside of ourselves. Two hours pass like this. Then the party departs for the downtown. Maria—the unicorn—grabs my arm.

"Come on," she says. "Follow me."

Together, we join the party—a moving caravan of drunkenness and disguise. Maria tugs me down Franklin Street, now blocked off from car travel and packed tight with Halloween costumes: Thor, Frankenstein, Marilyn Monroe, The Cat in the Hat. A string of identically dressed girls passes, holding hands as Russian dolls. We drink. We stumble up the intoxicated street to show off our costumes.

Maria pulls us onward, lowering her horn to clear a path. And when we have pushed far enough and the crowd begins to thin, we retrace our steps through the swaying sea of celebration. At streetside, we drink and watch the spectacle. The crowd thickens. When a college fraternity parades by in marching band regalia, we duck into a crowded bar and press to the counter for more beers that we then take outside, and when these are finished, Maria leans against me and tells me that she should go back soon, that she is tired.

We return to Jake's to retrieve our cars and before leaving, there is an awkward pause as we decide how to part.

"I've had a wonderful time," the unicorn says. "This was really a nice Halloween surprise."

"It was something kind of *magical*, I suppose."

She comes toward me and we kiss, turning my head sideways to negotiate the horn.

Maria scribbles her number on a slip of paper, and I promise to call.

"Soon. Very soon," I say as she settles into her car seat and drives away.

When I return to my apartment, it is late, yet I am not tired but feel rejuvenated. I play several albums, and when the last one spins, I listen to the quiet dark settle around me, soothing and palpable. I place my thin, pale hand upon my heart and feel its beat.

WINTER IS THE

CRUELEST SEASON

November 1996. I try to reassemble my life. The grandeur of teaching seeming lost, I accept a position as a bookseller for Barnes & Noble in Durham, and more books pass through my hands than I could hope to read in a lifetime. I work eight-hour shifts and in the evenings, hobbled and stiff, I soothe my ankles in warm bathwater. I prop them on pillows and try to sleep, but they keep me awake. Often they worsen and, with the drape of moonlight around me, I mix my factor; constrict the tourniquet on my arm; slip the needle into a raised blue line running underneath my skin; and infuse. Then I sleep.

To cure my lonesomeness, I call Maria and invite her to dinner. When I first see her again—the unicorn costume long discarded—her face glows and even in the dead of November she smells like the spring dew that settles upon the grass in the early morning. We eat well. We laugh heartily. And I am drawn closer to her. She isn't silly like some girls, nor a heavy drinker, and I feel immediately how she begins to fill up the hole inside me. Before parting, we kiss beneath the lamplight of her apartment.

"I'm glad you called me," she says before going.

"Me, too."

"So let's do this again sometime. Perhaps after the hectic Thanksgiving holiday."

"Yes, let's. I'll call you."

The week before Thanksgiving a snow starts in the early morning. I pour coffee and sneak out into a morning made immaculate by a theophany of white. The cold sun filters through the clouds, and I squint at the brightness as I crunch through the frozen landscape. The winter birds flit through the longleaf pines and dodge the slow drip of a thawing world with the trees standing as colossal black pillars against the white garland of snow. Soon the puddles will begin and make soft mud of the earth, but today is luminous, the sky crisp and as blue as the color of ink run from a pen.

While my friend travels during the holidays, his two cats stay with me. When he drops them off, I place Somali, the oldest, in my lap and he purrs and curls up next to me as I stroke his thick fur.

"You're a pretty kitty."

He jumps down and scampers off.

"We'll be fine," I promise my friend as he pays me. "Your kitties and I will get along just great."

When I sleep, the cats pounce on the bed and startle me. I get up and set them outside my door, but they mew and paw at it, so to quiet them, I shake food in their bowls and return to bed, but soon they are back scratching at my door. When I leave, they claw at the furniture, sleep on the countertops, and prance on the kitchen tables, so that when I return, I have to clean hair and paw marks from the tabletops and, for the furniture, I fasten double-sided tape to the leg corners. Then, after a few weeks, the smell of shit from neglected litter or from Somali's upset stomach that causes him to go wherever begins to permeate the apartment's blue air; its noxious fumes greet me when the door is unsealed and a vacuumed whoosh of stool and piss is discharged. I gag. I heave. I clean the litter. I clean the carpet, the sofa, the sitting chair. I disinfect the kitchen. I pet the kitties, and as I stoop low to stroke their fur, it pulls off in my hand and I notice it has also chunked off on the floor, on the couch, and on my bed. But I'm too tired to clean anymore and only have the energy to retrieve my factor from the fridge and to fall asleep, rise to work, to treat, and to fall asleep again. The air of life has gasped out of me. I'm weary. Tired. And just putter around as best I can.

The phone rings. It is dark outside, and I locate the sound near my bed.

"Hey, Son. How are you? It's Mom. Just checking in . . ."

"Mom," I say.

"You're not already in bed are you? It's only nine."

"Just tired is all. Long day at work."

"You sound perfectly exhausted. Why don't you come home for the weekend? Dad can cook you a steak and you can get some rest. Are you eating?"

"Of course I'm eating."

"What'd you have for supper?" Oh, Mom's sly.

"Supper? I had a late lunch."

"At the bookstore? Couldn't have been more than a sandwich." She pauses. "I think you should talk to Dr. Trum when you see him next week. Don't you see him next week?"

"No. My appointment's not for another month. I had to change it because of work."

"You shouldn't do that. You should go to the doctor first. I just read an article in *Time* about Dr. Ho and these new protease inhibitors and it sounds promising. Maybe you could ask the doctors about them? I know you had a rough time before, but medicine has come a long way. You have to try something." She stops. "Hello," she says.

"Yes, I'm still here. I need to sleep, Mom."

"Okay, Son. Just think about. And come see us. Can you come this weekend? I think your sister is coming. She can swing by and pick you up."

"No. I have to close Saturday."

"Can't somebody work your shift?"

"I work Sunday, too. I had to switch to get last Tuesday off for the ID doctor."

"Well, okay. I just think you should quit it all. Come home for a few months."

"I need to sleep," I say.

"Okay, okay," she says, getting my hint. "I mailed you some money today to help out. Use it to pay some of the bills, and go treat yourself to a nice meal somewhere. Don't you like the Olive Garden? Or what's that place you took us to with the really good fried chicken? Dips? Or something like that."

"Okay, Mom. Thanks. I appreciate it. You didn't have to do that."

When we hang up, I sleep soundly—at least until midnight when the cats wake me, mewing and jumping on my bed, reminding me that I forgot to feed them.

For several nights, I awake and my bed is soaked through. My shirt is wet. My boxers. My legs and arms. In the night, my whole body is a cloud of pouring rain and my bed a reservoir of perspiration. I wring out my clothes and drape them over the shower rod while I fish through my dresser drawers for dry clothing. My eyes are red-rimmed. My tongue thick and sticking dryly to the roof of my dry, dry mouth. Even water cannot help it.

"I cannot eat," I tell the doctor. "When I try to swallow, my throat closes off and I gag."

The ID doctor holds my tongue down with the depressor. "Yep. Esophagitis. The thrush has worsened. We can fix that with another drug that's a bit stronger, and you should have your appetite back and be able to eat within a few days. I'm worried about that since your weight is down to 116. That's pretty slim . . . Now more than ever, you need to eat." He passes his stethoscope along my chest as I breathe in, breathe out. "Have you been keeping up with your Pentamidine?"

"Yes. I haven't missed a dose since I started."

"Good. There's a little fluid in there, and I don't want that to grow into anything like PCP, so I'm putting you on an antibiotic to take care of that." He writes the prescriptions and passes this off to me. "Do you have any questions?"

I draw a hand up to my eyes. The doctor stands beside me and passes me tissue. "I'm scared. I'm really scared."

"There's a lot to be scared of," he says. "I won't lie to you about that. And I won't tell you that I know how you feel or what you're going through because I don't. I can't even imagine it. But I can promise you that we'll give you the best care possible. And, although it may not seem like it right now, I feel you're in a really good position for treatment. It looks like the protease inhibitors are an effective treatment, and once the FDA approves them, which should be any day now, my feeling is that you're going to respond." I calm and dry my hands along my jeans, smoothing the creases with damp palms. "Just take the prescriptions I've given you, and you'll feel better in a few days and I'm sure that fluid in your chest is just a little winter cold. It's not anything to worry over just yet." He starts gathering his things. "Call me whenever you feel like. I mean it."

When our visit ends, I feel weighed down. Even my crying is no solace. I gather myself and exit into the lobby, wearing a brave mask as if nothing is wrong.

At home, I gargle. I swallow. And I stick out my tongue to the mirror and see the thin coating of fungus and the trace of it spreading down my throat. My face is sallow and carved tight round my cheekbones; my skin pockets near the mouth as if tiny invisible gumballs press around my teeth; and my eyes are dark, brooding, and sunken deep in the sockets. I raise my shirt to show a chest that is all bone and arms that are thin flaps of flesh. A fragile peel of skin shrinks round my body as wet tissue to a hand. The mirror does not lie.

I drop my pants to expose my only plump tissue, and to make myself happy for a time, I play, and when the moment ends, my plumpness shrivels into a congruency with the rest of my body.

I cough. I spit out a winter phlegm, thick and viscous. Then I feel chilled. I notch up the thermostat. My nose drizzles. My head hurts. My stomach aches. I feel flushed.

"I think I'm going to die," I tell William on the phone.

"What? Are you sick?"

"I don't know. I don't know what's happening. I just feel sick and tired and tired from feeling sick and tired." I blow my nose on some tissue. I cry. "And I'm scared."

"I'm coming to see you. I'll be there tonight."

The hours pass as I wait for William's company. I huddle in my bed. I watch some TV. I pet the kitties. And when I hear footsteps outside, I spread the blinds to see if it's William, but, disappointed, I wait. When he finally arrives and I let him in, he surveys my apartment.

"Oh my God," he exclaims. "You have got to get this place cleaned up. How many people are living here?"

"Just me and the kitties."

"You shouldn't be taking care of them. Your place looks like a disaster, and it smells awful."

"I know. I'm too tired to clean it. I can't do it anymore. I just can't."

I cry. William sits beside me on the couch and puts a soft hand to my back.

"We'll get this place cleaned up. It's going to be okay."

He drives to Walmart and buys cleaning supplies, and when he returns, he scrubs and disinfects every corner of my small apartment while I stare vacantly out the window at the barren trees swaying in the cold breeze. And although the place soon smells as clean as the day when I first moved in, it is still just as blue.

Later, we purr along in William's car, steering the Orange County back roads. The stars pierce the cold and the moon dangles like a giant orb in the black sky. The farmland, blanketed in night, appears as ashen silhouettes of barnlots and fenceposts, while a thin run of wire sometimes catches a flicker of headlight as we pass.

"I don't know if you want any," William says, "but I brought some smoke for you. I really think it would ease your pain and help you eat something."

"So, if I do, are you going to use me for your legalization campaign? Is that it? I'm your medical marijuana case?"

"Funny . . . I'm just laying out the facts. The choice is yours."

"I don't think I've got much to lose, so, yeah."

William pulls off onto a side road where a lone lamppost illuminates bluely as he idles the car and packs the bowl.

"Just breathe in like it's a cigarette."

"But I never smoked a cigarette."

"Never . . . goddamn . . . Well, just breathe in and hold. Here, I'll light it for you."

"No, I can handle that. I've watched it plenty."

The lighter flares. I inhale.

"Maybe one more time," William says.

I inhale again. And then I cough uncontrollably.

"Okay, that's enough. Here . . . drink some of my soda."

He passes me his drink and William's car purrs on as time soon melds into ribbons of darkness; a tingle of warmth puffs me up and floats me in the car seat.

"Where are we?" I ask, looking out at a dark wood of nothing.

"I don't know," William says. "But we'll be somewhere eventually."

We motor on underneath the canopy of night. A mosaic of pasture scrolls by as we speed along a deserted road where the trees, blunted by winter, stretch their spindly tendrils toward the sky, the moon, the stars.

"See that," I say to William as the sparkle of city lights again envelops us. "Waffle House! I'm starving."

He pulls in, gets out, and walks around the parking lot as if lost.

"What are you doing? Let's go inside."

"All right. I was just trying to figure where we are. Do you know where we are?"

"What difference does it make? Let's eat."

Inside, we slide into a booth and a grizzled lady with large yellow teeth strides over to us.

"Whataya'll have?"

"Where are we?" William asks distractedly.

"This here's the Waffle House, Son."

Immediately, I begin to cackle uncontrollably. Oh, I'm laughing it up, holding my sides and feeling as my stomach tightens and starts to ache.

"Is he all right?" the waitress asks William. "Son, you all right?" she asks, eyeballing me.

"Yeah," I say, calming my laughter. "Yeah. I'm fine."

"What town is this?" William asks.

"Just outside of Burlington," the waitress says. "Where ya headin'?"

"Oh, nowhere really."

"Uh-huh." She taps her pen on her yellow pad. "So you and your skinny friend want somethin' to eat?"

"Oh, yes," I say. "Eggs. I want lots of eggs."

"Okay," the waitress says flatly. "Can you be more specific? How many and how ya want 'em?"

"Two," I say. "No. Three. Scrambled. And can I get some hash browns? Double hash browns. Scattered and smothered." I trail my finger down the menu. "Oh, oh. And a side of bacon. And some toast."

"It comes with toast."

"Oh, excellent. And a cup of coffee to drink."

She turns to William. "And for you?"

"Just coffee."

"Uh-huh. So you're not hungry and your skinny friend is just back from Auschwitz."

"Something like that," William says.

The waitress leaves and calls the order to the cook. William catches my attention.

"You gotta calm down," he says. "The whole place is watching you."

"Okay, okay . . . I'm being weally, weally quiet." I lower my head, peer about. "Are we hunting wabbit?" Another guffaw comes, and I can't stop laughing. William slinks into the booth as I let out an endless string of giggles.

"I'm better," I say, quieting myself. "I won't laugh like that again. I promise."

William rights himself and lights a cigarette, thumps the ash. "I know it's good for you, but damn . . . Why didn't you start in the car or something?" William glances around, puffs his cigarette, blows out smoke. "Good. Here comes your food. That'll shut you up."

A few days later, with William departed and me back in the work routine, I awake one night and race to the bathroom and pour my insides out. When it passes, I take my temp, but find I have none. Then the world dizzies, and I huff and gag over the toilet, while my head pounds terribly. Eventually, I return to my bed and place a damp cloth on my forehead, but then I must run for the bathroom again. And then again. And again.

By morning, it hasn't stopped, so I call the hospital clinic, and they are, of course, concerned.

"You should come in right away," Dr. Trum advises. "Headaches and vomiting trouble me."

Too dizzy to drive myself, I call my sister in Raleigh, and after her concern eases, she agrees to carry me to the hospital. A half hour later we are unable to find the emergency room; we blunder through hallways under construction and wander around, following handmade signs until we then wait for an elevator that has a star indicating "ER—2nd Floor." I lug around a small bucket just in case my stomach turns again.

"How's your head?" Anne asks worriedly. She has been in a panic since she picked me up and whisked me to the hospital.

"It's okay. I think it's passing. I'm not that worried right now."

"Well, I'm worried. You've been dizzy and throwing up since last night."

"You didn't tell Mom, did you?"

"No, but I felt like I should. She's going to be concerned for sure."

"Well, let's just wait and see what it is. It could just be a small cold. Mom would have gone bonkers if I told her. That's why I called you instead. Besides, you're closer living in Raleigh."

"Gee, thanks."

The door opens and there stands Maria, the elevator's only passenger. It is an awkward moment when we recognize one another. She wraps her white coat around herself and moves from the door for us to come in.

"What floor?" she asks. She gives my sister a thorough looking over and although I can sense her misinterpretation, I am too ill to correct her.

"Two." I lean against the wall. Sweat beads on my forehead. "I forgot you worked here."

"Yep. I do." She places a strand of hair behind her ear. "I haven't seen you in a while. Thought you were going to call."

"I guess I've been busy. The holidays, you know."

I want to add more, but we ride in silence, watching as the floor lights change from 1 to 2, and as the door opens and my sister and I exit the elevator, I turn to Maria.

"I'll call you." But my words are crippled before they leave my mouth.

"Okay, but you don't have to say that." She smiles. The door closes.

"Who was that?" Anne asks.

"Maria. We went out and I was suppose to call her back. I never did."

"Oh." Anne laughs. "What luck."

At the emergency room, they page Dr. Trum and when he arrives, he checks my lungs, which are relatively clean, and shines a light in my pupils to check my response.

"It looks okay," he says, "but I want to do a CAT scan on you just the same. Headaches and vomiting are not good signs for hemophiliacs. Head traumas are too deadly to play around with." My breath stills. "It is probably nothing, but it's always best to err on the side of caution."

For the CAT scan, I lie flat on the steel-cold bed while a dye is fed into my veins. The electric lights hum, the doughnut contraption whirs, and the bed slides through the portal. My heart beats with the worry of what may be found: a tumor, a slow bleed in my cranium. Nothing I imagine brings me any comfort.

Afterwards as Anne and I wait in the lobby, Anne twists her nervous hands together, twirls fingers through her hair.

"I think we should call Mom. This sounds serious."

"No, let's wait for the results. Then we'll either have the good news or the *really, really* bad news."

"This isn't funny. Why are you making this into a joke?"

"I'm not. I'm really not. I just don't know how else to be."

Dr. Trum ambles down the hallway with the films and kneels beside us, his tie swinging as a pendulum between his knees.

He balls his knuckles and knocks them atop my scalp. "There's nothing wrong with that head of yours. I think you just had a touch of something. Not that that's good for someone with your immunity, but well . . . it could have been worse. I want to give you something for nausea, and I'll call you later with the results from your blood tests, but I doubt if we'll find anything there. You've already stopped throwing up, haven't you?"

"I have."

"That's good. Maybe this thing has passed." He stands and stares down at me. "There's hope on the horizon," he says. "Hang in there."

When we return to my apartment, Anne falls into the couch and sweeps her eyes around my apartment while I get us drinks. The cats run through the room and disappear again. Then they are in front of us and Anne reaches down to pet them. Ice clinks in our glasses as we sit in the calm aftermath.

"Can we call Mom now?" Anne asks.

"Yeah. Now is fine. It's over."

She goes in my room and comes out a long time later.

"Mom wants to talk to you. She's on the phone."

I pick up the receiver.

"Hey, Mom."

"Come home and rest," she pleads. "Anne says you look terrible. We're all worried sick, and it's no good you staying up there by yourself like that. What are you trying to prove? It's Christmas for God's sake. Why can't you come home?"

"I can't. I'm not trying to prove anything. I'm just trying to live, to pay the bills, to survive. And I can't come home. I have to work tomorrow." I breathe quietly on the line and listen to Mom trying to hold in her tears. "Don't cry, Mom. It's not that bad. Please, don't cry."

"Just come home, Son. Can't you do that for us at Christmas? Just come home. That's all we want."

COCKTAILS

January 1997. When the new year begins, it is as any other year in winter: cold and frigid. Outside, ice freezes to the sprouts of twigs and to the sprigs of grass long since frostbitten, and the cold wind chaps the ground. Inside, my life feels frozen. I awake, eat a breakfast of cold cereal, and read a few pages of a novel; the rumble of cats is gone—their owner picked them up a few days ago—and now I am here alone.

I let myself out into the chill morning for an appointment with the ID doctor. And when the exam room door swings open and startles me from my little nap, I rise and catch the hint of a smile on his face. He leans against the wall, folds his arms across his chest, and studies me with his gaze.

"It's time," he says. "The Crixivan is approved, and I want you to start this protease inhibitor right away with two other drugs. A cocktail, we're calling it. How do you feel about that?"

"I'll take it. I'll do whatever is required."

He writes out the prescriptions, and as he passes the slips of paper into my hopeful hands, I recall the failure of AZT, but Crixivan *is* something I say, puffing up hope. Along with Crixivan I take d4T and 3TC—names that seem invented by George Lucas—and when I fill them at the hospital pharmacy, and when Crixivan arrives from a pharmacy on the West Coast—the only current distributor of this protease inhibitor—I squeeze the bottles in my hands, close my eyes in silent hope, and begin the cocktail treatment.

For the d4T and 3TC, I must take one pill twice a day with food; the Crixivan, however, requires three pills ingested three times a day at *exactly* eight hours apart. Consequently, Crixivan punctuates my days. When my midnight alarm goes off, I wake to take the Crixivan that I keep by my bedside, and after I sleepily choke down the large pills with several gulps of water, I reset the alarm for eight when I must awake for work and must also take my next dose. And when 4:00 P.M. arrives and I am caught on the book floor, my watch's alarm going off, I must discreetly excuse myself to the water fountain and swallow my three pills in as inconspicuous a manner as possible. And so it is done.

The months pass. This schedule becomes as familiar to me as each pill's size and weight, which I can register by their feel in the palm of my hand when I reach out for them in the dark or snag them with my fingers when they become buried in the deep pocket of my jeans. The Crixivan is a large capsule, the d4T smaller and also a capsule, and the 3TC tiny like a diamond-cut aspirin.

Naturally, Mom is hopeful about this treatment. She mails me an article about Dr. Ho and protease inhibitors, and as I curl on my couch with my coffee, having just swallowed my morning doses of all three meds, I read the interview about this modern-age Merlin and his potion for the HIV world. I cling to this as a man must grasp rope when hung from a building ledge, a cavernous drop.

In late April, my alarm wakes me and I refill my water glass, take the d4T, the 3TC, and the three pills of Crixivan—and I amble for the toilet on my stiff ankles as the sprinkle of weak sunlight filters through my blinds. A gripping pain seizes me in the back. I gnaw my tongue and curse out loud for the internal burning; I brace against the wall while my knees buckle and drop me to the floor. I stand again, aim, then out pisses blood.

Oh, fuck. I'm bleeding.

Although I'm a bleeder, seldom do I see blood. Instead I witness its effects in the swelling of a joint, in the stretching of skin, and in its pain. I calm myself by taking deep breaths. I hike up my boxers and return to bed, thinking of what to do. First, I cancel work, telling them that I have an emergency, and then I call the hospital to say that I'm on the way.

In the emergency room, a hematologist waits for me. He is a young man from a foreign country who explains to me that he is in America for a year to study medicine. In his country, he says as we settle into an examination room, no one really knows what hemophilia is, nor do they understand how to treat it. I am lucky here in America, he says starting an IV. In America, he says, they take care of you. In his homeland, he says, boys just like myself hobble about with swollen knees and they must drag themselves through the hot sands of his country because they go so long without medicine. And I imagine it: my other.

Turning his attention to me, he says, "We are going to run a great many tests on you and will see what the results give us."

"But what do you think it is?"

"I cannot say."

"But can't you guess? Is it bad?"

"I cannot say," he repeats, helping me into the bed and checking the drip on my IV. "But I think it is probably something with your kidneys. Perhaps a stone or some very bad bruising. But really, I cannot say."

When he leaves, I call Mom, and she tells me in a breathless panic that she is in the car and on her way and will be here soon. And when I try to reach Dad at the plant, the operator returns and explains that Mr. Smoak isn't answering his phone or his pages.

"Listen. This is an emergency and I need to speak with him immediately. Does your plant have a smoking area?"

"Yes."

"Try there and tell him it's his son."

I wait. The hall nurse comes in and introduces herself and says that an orderly is on his way to take me to X-ray. Then, as she leaves, Dad picks up the phone line. He coughs and is breathing fast from what I imagine to have been his brisk run from the outdoor smoking patio to the nearest phone.

"Son. Son, are you okay? What's happened?"

"I'm in the hospital, Dad."

"Oh goddamn."

"I feel fine, but there's blood in my urine."

"Do they know what's causing it?" He coughs.

"No. Not yet. They've got me scheduled for an ultrasound and an X-ray later, and then they'll know, but they're thinking it's my kidneys."

"Have you called your mother?"

"She's on the way."

"All right." Dad catches his breath, coughs heavy. "I'll be there quick as I can."

Later, everyone is in my room. Mom and Dad grip nervous hands together; Dr. Trum arrives with the medical student; the ID doctor ushers in his team; and the urologist enters, followed by his three shadows. The senior doctors talk while his understudies record notes on their clipboards. Soon they form a horseshoe around my bed. Mom, Dad, and I look on as Dr. Trum begins to speak.

"We're pretty sure it's your Crixivan," he says. "You've got kidney stones from it, and I've worked with the urologist to develop a plan of action."

"The Crixivan? What am I going to do about that?"

"We're going to start you on another protease inhibitor, Viracept, imme-diately. It has just been approved and should be, we hope, equally as effective as the Crixivan but, of course, without giving you those stones. You can't go back on the Crixivan. It's too much of a risk. Unfortunately, stones are one of its side effects." He looks away to the clock, then back. "Of course, we'd hoped you'd be in the clear on that one, but, well . . . you're not."

"These stones," the urologist says as he holds up an X-ray film to the light, "are not like other stones." He passes the film to his shadows, who examine my photo. "They are crystal in form and consequently have jagged edges. And, more importantly, they are too big to pass in your urine. If they did pass, I assure you . . . it would be quite painful." I imagine something like a shard of glass slicing its way down my urethra. "As you can see, and especially given your hemophilia, we must get rid of that stone before it cuts you even more." The shadows scribble furiously, this being, I imagine, good stuff for them. "Normally we would use sonic vibrations to break apart the stone, but that, I'm afraid, will simply cause more bleeding." Here, I envision several thousand shards of glass sluicing my urethra, snaring on tissue, and furrowing rows of deep vermilion. "I've talked with Dr. Trum and we agree that it's best if we go through your urethra and retrieve the stone and bring it out safely."

Oh horror!

"Good God," my father belts out. "I can't handle this. I'm leaving for a smoke." He rises from his seat, grabs his cigarettes, and shoves them into his shirt pocket as he spreads apart the doctors and makes his way for the exit.

"Will I be awake? Will I feel what's happening to me?" I ask.

"No. We'll put you under while we insert a tube and you shouldn't feel a thing," the urologist says, addressing my mother and me. "We will, however, have to leave a stent in to help the healing which, I'm afraid, will have to be removed while you're awake, but that's only a little discomfort."

"And we'll keep you factored up throughout the whole procedure," Dr. Trum chimes in. "We'll be sure your levels stay up to stop any bleeding."

"What about my job?"

"I think you're going to need at least two to three weeks off."

"Oh, I can't do that. I don't have vacation days and I've used up all my sick leave."

"Forget about your job," Mom interrupts. "You need to get better. This isn't the time to think about that bookstore. It couldn't give two hoots about you."

I don't argue with her. On the verge of tears, she blows her nose to distract herself. "Okay," I say. "Okay."

Then, the plan in place, the physicians file out uniformly.

In the evening, Mom drives out to find us some food worth eating. Dad and I sit with the TV on.

"Son," Dad says during a commercial. "I know you don't want to hear this, but I think you should just move back home. You can't keep working at that job like you are. Your kidneys are going to need time to heal and you've just started those cocktails and your mom and I have talked and we just think you need to rest and give that stuff a chance to work." Dad rubs his mustache and stretches out his lanky legs. "Anne says that you've been writing short stories or something like that. She says you gave her something you did and she thought it was pretty good. Maybe you should just come home and do something like that. It would keep you from being so bored while you tried to get back on your feet. You need rest, Son. We all can see it. You're too thin. And, well, you're just too run down."

"I'll think about it."

"Think hard, Son. You've got insurance through COBRA and that's good for over a year, so there's no reason for you to stay up here. No reason at all. Work will always be there for you. Trust me on that. But your home and a place to rest and recover won't be."

Outside the sky starts to purple and is soon stricken in darkness. We sleep.

The following morning, I am wheeled into the operating room. The anesthesia burns into my vein, but then I remember nothing. And when I wake, I am back in my room, the TV is on, and Mom and Dad are propped in chairs beside me.

"They said it went fine," Mom says when she notices me rousing. She walks over to my bed and brushes hair from my face. "How do you feel?"

"Like shit, really. And I'm scared as hell to use the bathroom."

Soon, a nurse comes in and changes out my factor bag, and I watch as it begins to drips down my IV. She takes my temp, checks my blood pressure, empties my bloody urinal, and is gone. I sleep. I wake and glance over to Mom and Dad, who still sit in their chairs beside me.

"Okay," I say. "I've had enough. I'm moving home."

For another week, I lie in that hospital bed and every time I pee, I brace myself for the pain and I cross my fingers for clear, unbloodied urine. At first, my urine is dark like a thick merlot, but then, as the days go on, it begins to lighten and then is pink and, eventually, is clear, leading to my discharge.

Having resigned from Barnes & Noble and made arrangements to break the lease on my blue, blue apartment, I return home. Mom and Dad drive their cars up and load my things, and then we leave, carrying my body home to rest. Outside, the roadside pastures bloom around me and it seems that spring will inter me as we glide over the Uwharries' rolling hills. The dogwood trees are just beginning to flower and they group about the fronts of fading farmhouses, their brilliant white bracts open for pollination. The pines and the rich-green cedars lord over the clover and crabgrass which presses through the thaw. Overhead, a troop of starlings flies in the dull blue sky, and when we park in our drive, they seem to come near, alighting in the yard before lifting off in an ocean of caws.

At the house, I help as best I can to unload the cars and U-Haul, but, still recovering, still worried I might piss blood again, I hang back and watch the furniture, boxes, and household accoutrements pass by as Mom and Dad transport them from U-Haul to bedroom and then return for another arm-load. At every third or fourth trip, Dad pauses for a smoke and then begins again. And when the sun begins to sag under the flat ceiling of sky and the U-Haul is empty and returned, we gather at the table for a meal, and then, all of us heavy with fatigue, we disperse to our rooms.

I lie on my bed and feel a great weight upon me. I am worn out. I have failed again, and, at twenty-five, am returned home. I breathe out; my heart flaps in a chest of bone.

Through my window, daylight constricts and soon a ribbon of moonlight casts its onion color on the stacks of boxes clustered about the room. I rise, root through one, and, finding a book, begin reading and let its fiction eclipse my reality.

RECOVERY

MAY 1997. I BEGIN ANOTHER COCKTAIL THERAPY WHERE VIRACEPT replaces Crixivan, and time is again measured in the eight-hour intervals my medicine requires, this only punctuated by the meals my mom prepares: breakfast becomes lunch becomes dinner. I sleep. I read. It is a soft living, an inviting picture. Yet my leg and ankle joints remain swollen, and mornings I am an ungreased machine. Arthritis having settled in, I am feeling what hemophilia does to a body as it ages. But it is not as bad as it has been, for now I am able to rest.

My hometown is just as I have remembered it: quiet with nothing happening. The three o'clock factory shift changes are as punctual as the noontime fire whistle that I can hear drifting to me over the vacant pasture and the few brick homes between the siren and me. I will pause from my reading only long enough for my mind to connect that low moan with something that exists in the real world. And then it fades away. I read more.

Spring passes into summer.

The daytimes are searing hot, but the evenings are a pleasant treasure. Louise, who earns a few coins in the local workshop program, also helps punctuate my day by her arrival home by bus at five. She lumbers down the stairs to my room, peeks her head through my door—her Down eyes big and brown behind thick glasses—and says, "Hey," in a short thick language that is her own.

"Hey, Louise," I will answer. "Did you have a good day at the workshop?"

"Good day," she says.

And then I will bookmark my read and follow her upstairs, for I know by her arrival that the sun has just lowered itself behind the tall longleaf pines and that the whole of our back deck is now shaded. The deck is a new addition. A wall was knocked out, the deck was raised. And now, being above the low Chinese elms in our backyard, I can look past the fence line that hedges our property and into the pasture due west. Here, the sun descends.

I take my coffee with cream and sugar and watch the sunset view from this deck. By the time I begin my second cup, the final sunbursts flare into the horizon and then soften into a strata of purple that cloaks the yard and its unseen crickets in plum darkness. The sparks of fireflies flash here, then there, then here again—their formless floating glows filling up the darkness. And with the stars out, the moon up, Mom has supper prepared. I eat, have another coffee, and read more until my tired eyes tell me they need rest.

Soon I begin swimming at the YMCA. I undress and slip my legs into the suit. I dip into the indoor pool's cool water. Beside me, a man adjusts his cap, his goggles. He is hairy like a bear, and he pushes off from the side, makes a heavy kick and swims. I swim. He swims faster. My arms grow heavy. My lungs ache. And it is much too far to the other side. When I reach it, I hold onto the ledge gasping, wheezing heavily. The bear beside me tucks and shoves off from his second lap. I go another length, and, dizzy with exhaustion, I feel as if I have swum an ocean. My head spins. I gasp. My heart pounds itself against my thin ribs, and I hold my chest to keep it from bursting out.

I get out, dry myself off, and watch as the bear keeps at it. *Soon, I'll swim like him*, I think. *Soon.*

When the cool breezes begin to blow in the fall, I return to see Dr. Trum. I feel healthier and think that my quiet convalescence at home has improved me, but my counts will tell the truth. They are always a sobering marker of my reality. Dr. Trum walks in, slides my folder open on his table.

"How are those cocktails doing?" he asks.

"I'm tolerating them. I'm not missing any doses."

"That's good. That's good." He edges closer to me, smiles fully for what I think is the first time. I notice a silver cap on his rear tooth. "Take a look at this," he says pointing to a sheet with numbers.

"Two hundred and three," I read.

"Now this." He points again.

"Undetectable."

He wheels backwards, crosses his feet, raises his arms and holds them behind his head. "That first is your CD4s going up, and that last is your viral load going down. Now what do you think about that?"

I can't hide my grin. My Merlin has come through after all with his healing potion.

"That sounds like damn good news to me. That's the best news you've ever given me, Doc."

"I'm glad I could give it. Doctors never really like giving the bad news, you know. You should take this bit of good news about your recovery and gloat a while. It's been a long time coming."

That evening as I stroll up and down the road before my house, my heart is a globe of happiness. I feel unshackled and alive. The lights glow here and there in the windows of neighbors' homes. Fireflies flicker and hover before the boughs of dark trees, and a woodpecker burrows into cedar and underneath him a cricket sings the sun down. Although the air is lethargic and redolent of late summer, it is full of humming life.

"Call me, too, Ishmael," I yell out to the slip of moon just visible in the navy night, "for I have survived myself."

All my family comes and eats with me in our house, and they share in my happiness.

"We really couldn't be more pleased," Mom says with wet eyes as we hold our wine glasses up for a toast.

"I will now live a hundred and forty years!"

"Here! Here!"

And later, I flatten a blank sheet of paper across my desk. I fill the vacant night with my words and exhaust myself with the stars. It is in this manner that I begin another kind of recovery. I write:

When Jimmy was ten, HIV came to him through a blood transfu-sion, but neither the doctor, nor his mother, nor his father knew this until Jimmy was thirteen. And when the doctor uncovered the virus in Jimmy's blood, he immediately phoned Jimmy's mother to tell her of this sad news. She stretched the phone cord across their kitchen, and, while she talked, she stared vacantly out the half-sized window over the sink which looked into their acre backyard. Standing on his toes, Jimmy had just grown tall enough to peek out this window, and he arched up to discover what his mother saw there. Winter coming, the leaves had fallen from the shade trees, and he could see far into the pasture to the cows which stood gumming grass idly in the cooling breeze, underneath the pewter sun.

His mother looked down to Jimmy who was pulling on her shirt, trying to gain her attention.

"Now, go away, Son," she said. "Mommy has some business to attend to. Go play in the yard." And she waved her hand as if shoo-ing a fly.

Jimmy left and hid himself on the nearby stairs until his mother finished her conversation. "No," he heard her cry out. "No. It's not true." Then she slammed the phone back on its rest and ran down the hallway past Jimmy, hidden on the stairs. He heard the thwack of her bedroom door and the hollow echo it made throughout their tiny hall-way. Then Jimmy heard a great sorrow wailing from that room.

His sisters ventured from their rooms, and they peered quizzically at the closed door. In Jimmy's house, they never kept their doors shut, for they were a family.

"What's going on?" Lisa asked. Her fifth-grade hair twined in pig-tails, she reasoned with the dark wood grain of her mother's shut door, scrutinized its unusual closing with her kid eyes.

"I don't know," Jimmy said.

Being as still as pond water, they congregated on the stairtop and listened to their mother's tears.

"Mommy cries," Constance said in her thick Down tongue. "She upset."

They hovered there for some time, played the short shags of carpet in their fingers, and peered down the hallway to their mother's closed door. Time passed.

"I'm going down there," Lisa said.

And she did. She crawled silently on all fours; only the quiet scruff of her knees across carpet sounded in the house. At the door, she stopped and Jimmy saw as she cupped her ear to it and then raised her hand as if to knock. But she dropped it quickly and scurried back.

"She's still crying," Lisa said, panting softly, quietly. "I can hear it through the door." They all gazed down the hall.

"Mommy still cries," said Constance, rocking cross-legged on her haunches.

They waited.

An hour later, their father came home from work, and the three siblings rushed him at the door and explained that something was wrong with their mother. He went in, shut the door behind him, and they waited, again.

Much later, he came out and woke the children asleep on the stairs. The house was dark. The outside was dark.

"Are you kids hungry?" he asked.

"Yes," they said, rubbing their soft eyes of sleep.

"We're going to eat out, tonight," he said. "How's McDonald's sound?"

He talked not so much to his son and daughters as to the ceiling. He blew into his pristine white handkerchief, wiped his nose, and cleared his eyes, which were wet with tears, and then placed the monogrammed cloth back into his pocket. Then the children knew something was wrong. Their father was upset, which seldom happened, and their mother wasn't cooking, which only happened when they traveled.

"Mommy going to be all right?" Constance asked, pointing her petite finger toward the room, the door still closed.

"She'll be just fine," their father said. "She just found out some really bad news is all. Both of us found out some bad news."

"What kind of news?" Lisa asked.

"It's nothing for you to worry about," the father said, pulling the

children to him. He towered above them like a statue. "Nothing to worry about." And they hugged. And their father cried some more.

"Are you ready to eat?" he asked, breaking their long, mournful embrace.

"Yes."

So, they piled into the family car, now thinking about hamburgers and crisp fries while their mother stayed, still shut up and crying behind her closed door.

When they returned, she had the tea glasses iced and filled, the napkins folded round, and the plates set out at their places, and none mentioned her tears as they ate their meal in silence.

THE OPEN DOOR

1998. There is but one thing left to do. I find the scrap of paper given me so long ago and dial the number. The phone rings in the receiver. She answers.

"Hey, Maria. This is Shelby."

And I can feel her smile at the other end, for it is my own.

Often I've thought about her and have wondered what happened, but I never called. For me, Maria was a travesty of timing. Then I had nothing of myself to share with her. I consider how my life has depended so much on timing. My factor invented the same year I was born, that's timing. My health falling in dangerous decline just when protease inhibitors and cocktail therapies swooped in to sustain me, that's timing. And now, calling Maria just as I'm beginning to feel the other parts of my life falling into place . . . perhaps this is timing.

"And where have you been?" she asks.

"Recovering," I say.

"And just who was that girl you were pulling around the hospital that last time I saw you?"

"Oh," I say laughingly. "That was my sister and that is just another long story that you'll have to endure someday."

We make plans and when the upcoming weekend of our date arrives, I

197

drive to Chapel Hill and spot Maria waiting under the restaurant's awning, her coat wrapped snug about her.

"Wow," she says when I near. "You've really filled out."

I run my hand over my chest and puff it out a bit.

"It's the swimming, I believe. The plentiful rest I've had while at home."

"Well, you look great."

"I'm even better now."

We pull ourselves together, and it is good to feel her next to me. At dinner, I explain about my past. And when I tell her about my HIV, she never flinches.

"So now that you're better, what are you going to do next?"

"Well, since you ask . . . I think I'm going to write a memoir."

"Humph." She sips her wine. I mine. "That's like an autobiography, right?"

"Yeah, I guess."

"Well, what's the difference?"

"I'm not sure. Maybe it's like *sofa* and *couch*. The same."

"Well, I think it'll make a great story." She sips again. "Think I'll be in it?"

"Maybe. I haven't gotten to the ending yet, so there's a possibility."

Outside, the summer is young and warms us both, and as I stroll the street I walked in less happier times, I feel that sick tug in my gut. I see the coffee shop where I drank away my fatigue and the road I took every day to Aster Elementary and then to Barnes & Noble. But Maria turns to me, takes my hand.

"Are you okay?" she asks. "You seem melancholy."

"I'm okay. Just remembering is all."

"Don't worry about it. That's the past. This is the future." And she smiles again, tugs like a child at my arm.

And later that night she tells me she's glad we ran into each other again, happy we both had a year of getting better.

We sip more wine, shed our clothes in the coolness of her apartment room.

"I'm not just some girl," she says, our flesh bodies cooling off from passion, from heat.

"I never thought you were."

And at night when we sleep, her legs jerk and jump and rouse me from my slumber. I wake her, calling her Rabbit for the fields I think she must skip through in dreams.

"Where were you hopping to?" I stroke her supple back, her resting body.

"Nowhere. I'm going nowhere if that's okay with you."

She drifts back off, her slender arms around me.

The next day, we go for a picnic, passing through the valleys, groves, hills, and fields before pulling off on an open stretch of country road. We hike down a small ravine and sit upon the rocks by the shallow riverside while around us the melodious birds sing. It is an unreal moment, one that is more something one would read in a poem, and less something that would happen. And yet it has.

When the warm sun goes down around our picnic, we spread ourselves on a blanket, lie flat against our backs, and stare up into the night sky to trace the constellations with our young fingers. I spy the Milky Way of stars, which are a hazy cluster against the jet-black dark. We lie there so long that soon clouds come and blow over our view of the night sky. And rain follows. The sweet scent of summer rain pours upon us, making puddles of the ground, while we gather our things and dash for the car.

As we drive away, a tumultuous sky sparks rods of lightning, and the earth smells serene. The wet swish of my tires clicks off the miles as I speed along open road. The cool night drifts damply through my down-rolled window while beside me Maria has already fallen asleep. She is comfortable and at peace, as am I.

Merging onto the interstate, a passing eighteen-wheeler disrupts my tranquility, plowing through the rainy dark, spewing spray in my path and roaring loudly. I let it pass. The taillights blur across my windshield as the semi merges back into my lane and dusts my drive with upturned mist, the truck's red flash stark against the black-wet road, the black-wet sky.

The storm sparks: a gentle flicker over a clean-washed road. My enormous heart beats on. I breathe in. Breathe out. Breathe in. Breathe.

ACKNOWLEDGMENTS

I'D LIKE TO THANK MY WIFE, VICKY, FOR HER UNENDING AND unquestionable support and love; all my friends who became unwitting characters in this book, all those who, for one reason or another didn't, but who I know I can lean on just the same; the teachers who've guided me to this path; the countless caregivers (especially the UNC Hemophilia and Thrombosis Center) who've kept me in the game of life; the health care professionals at Caremark and BioRx who've assured that I've gotten my medicines, maintained my insurance, and stayed in relative comfort and peace of mind; PSI whose contribution in paying my insurance premiums in times of need is inestimable; PEN American for their generous and needed grant; and my family for supporting me through illness and health, especially to Mom and Dad who, instead of propping me in front of a TV when I was ill, gave me books to read and showed me a whole world of ideas—a place I just might fit into.